WILD RIDE HOME

WILD RIDE HOME

Love, Loss, and a Little White Horse:

A Family Memoir

CHRISTINE HEMP

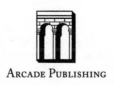

ARCADE PUBLISHING

Copyright © 2020 by Christine Hemp

All rights reserved. No part of this book may be reproduced in any manner without the express written consent of the publisher, except in the case of brief excerpts in critical reviews or articles. All inquiries should be addressed to Arcade Publishing, 307 West 36th Street, 11th Floor, New York, NY 10018.

Arcade Publishing books may be purchased in bulk at special discounts for sales promotion, corporate gifts, fund-raising, or educational purposes. Special editions can also be created to specifications. For details, contact the Special Sales Department, Arcade Publishing, 307 West 36th Street, 11th Floor, New York, NY 10018 or arcade@skyhorsepublishing.com.

Arcade Publishing® is a registered trademark of Skyhorse Publishing, Inc.®, a Delaware corporation.

Visit our website at www.arcadepub.com.

10 9 8 7 6 5 4 3 2

Library of Congress Cataloging-in-Publication Data is available on file.

Cover design by Erin Seaward-Hiatt
Cover art by Bénédicte Gelé

Printed in the United States of America

Hardcover ISBN: 978-1-950691-24-1
Paperback ISBN: 978-1-951627-78-2
Ebook ISBN: 978-1-950691-33-3

Parts of this manuscript (in slightly different forms) have appeared in the *Iowa Review*, *Fourth River*, and *Writing on the Edge* at the University of California, Davis. Other sections were aired on National Public Radio's *Living on Earth* and posted on *This I Believe*. Portions have also been awarded a Washington State Arts Commission Artist Trust Fellowship for Literature, a Barbara Deming/Money for Women Grant, a Donald Murray Award for Nonfiction, an Annie Dillard Award from *Bellingham Review*, a residency at Vermont Studio Center, and a first runner-up for the Iowa Award for Literary Nonfiction.

for my family, both here and there

We Manage Most When We Manage Small
... Making safety in the moment. This touching
home goes far. This fishing in the air.
— Linda Gregg

⮂Author's Note⮀

DEAR READER: I HAVE TRIED to be vigilant about the facts of my story and am painfully aware that memory is a sticky business. My interpretation of events will undoubtedly differ from another's, and time can be elastic, too. I have done my best to stay true to chronology, but some passages are compressed to serve the story. The only factual changes I deliberately made were the names and details of several people and places to protect their privacy. Other than that, a memoir is always a matter of selective memory (what's left out remains as potent as what is included), and I found I had to succumb to this story's own particular power. I write to keep fear and sorrow at bay. I write to celebrate what I've found. I write to find out more. Finally, I write out of love, for even after all these years, I still believe my mother's words that echo in my earliest memories: "It will all work out."

—Christine Hemp
Olympic Peninsula, Washington State
2020

Table of Contents

PART I:
LAND OF ENCHANTMENT

Chapter 1.

⮌ *Pressure and Release* ⮌

A BALD EAGLE SKIMS ALONG the bluff where windblown Douglas firs, their exposed roots like talons, grip the eroding cliff. Gulls circle and warn the bird of prey not to come too close. One hundred fifty feet below, the Salish Sea crashes and stretches west to the Pacific.

I arrive on foot with an empty water bucket just as the morning sun spills across the field. Near the meadow gate a small, white horse and two mules are dozing. The horse's delicate head flies up when he hears me coming. He nickers and nods. I sneak a lead rope around his neck (no time for hide-and-seek today) and brush his bright coat while he picks up a stick and waves it in the air as if conducting an orchestra. "Come on, Buddy—" I tell him, "We have places to go." I toss the brush into the bucket along with my sandwich, skinny him out the gate so the mules won't escape, then tack him up with an old bridle I'd saved since childhood. He gnaws at the bit, dancing in place. After sidling him over to a sawhorse, I jump up with one hand clutching both reins and a long hank of white mane, slip my leg over his bare back, and carefully lift the bucket in my other hand. As my weight settles, the bucket rattles and Buddy rears and skitters so frantically I have to drop it. So much for supplies. We head off down the road, Buddy's legs in a whir, his nostrils wide, my heart beating fast.

Buddy isn't the only cause for apprehension (he shies at everything from plastic bags to rabbits); it's the thought of seeing horse people again. My teenage 4-H horse-show days return, and, even in middle age, insecurity rises like a warm flood. I can certainly ride this snappy gelding—I've been doing that all summer—but reentry into a world of "the right tack" or "registered" horses spooks me more than Buddy with the bucket.

After the mile ride to the Fairgrounds, the first person we see is a woman in shiny boots and breeches unloading a black horse from a trailer. I try not to think of my scratched-up logging boots, my red-and-gray fishing hat, or the car-wash brush I'd been using to groom Buddy, now left behind in the bucket along with my lunch.

"Hi!" the woman says. "Cute little gray Arabian! Hey, if you need anything, I've got buckets and such."

"Oh, thanks!" I say, "Yes, I could use a water bucket—I had to leave mine behind."

She sets one near an empty stall. "I'll see you up there!" she smiles and points to where people are gathering. I fill the bucket, slip Buddy into the stall, and hurry to the outdoor arena. A compact man in jeans, tennis shoes, and a wide-brimmed, water-stained Australian Outback hat is talking to a cluster of women. A half-smoked cigarette hangs from his fingers. When I approach, he turns to me, his blue-gray eyes clear and welcoming. "Hi," he says, holding out a strong, square hand. "I'm Ken."

A young woman leads her bay Morgan into the arena, and Ken asks her horse's name. "Tika," she says and stops next to the mare's shoulder while the rest of us retreat to the bleachers. The mare tenses as the woman mounts.

"Hmmmm," Ken says. "Why don't you walk her out." The horse steps in a perfect circle, turning with agility and arching her neck like a professional dressage horse. I think of Buddy's head carriage—wild and high—and wonder how this Morgan has come to be so compliant. "Looks like she's been told what to do so much she can't even make a decision on her own," Ken says. To me the mare looks alive and full of zest, but Ken sees something else.

"See her eyes?" Ken turns to us. "She is so afraid of doing the wrong thing, she can't move out freely. She's packed in there tight." I begin to see it. The horse's eyes are wary and her shoulders tremble slightly, a shadow of sweat forming on her chest.

"Tami," Ken says gently, "Your horse may seem like a safe horse to ride, but someday she may lose her cool over something really small."

I wait for Ken to speak about seat, Tami's hands, or her position. But riding is never discussed. He focuses only on the horse.

"We need to uncover what's in there," Ken says, "and give this mare the opportunity to be in partnership, not fear." Ken lays his hand on the horse's neck. "What this horse needs is confidence." Ken's language is completely new to me. No one talked this way in my 4-H group when I'd had my childhood horse, Lightfoot, or when I'd ridden other horses since. It was as if he were telling me something I knew but hadn't ever been able to articulate.

When I go to check on Buddy at the break, I'm horrified to discover him weaving back and forth in his stall, his head swaying, his eyes in a panic. Buddy's owner, my neighbor Fred, had told me that Buddy had done the same thing with him. That's why he'd moved him out of a small paddock into the big field on Henry Street with two mules for company. I'd never seen Buddy in a stall before—he and the mules ran loose in the meadow—and the weaving disturbed me. Why had I brought Buddy to this training clinic without asking Fred? Was I in over my head? Horses were fraught with worry and crisis. I knew plenty about that.

Afraid someone might see Buddy's neurosis, I quickly put on his bridle, lead him to the arena, and stand with him outside the gate. He rubs my shoulder with his nose and fidgets with the bit, sometimes trying to reach into my pocket.

When the group breaks for lunch Ken walks over and says, "Are you coming to eat? There's pizza for everyone." I perk up at the sound of food, but I can't think of what I'd do with Buddy.

"Oh, I think I'll just wait here. My horse doesn't seem to like the stall…," I say, lying about Buddy being mine, and hoping Ken won't think me an idiot that he can't be stabled.

"Well, that's okay. If he doesn't like it, then don't put him in there." Ken pointed over my shoulder. "Why not just turn him loose in the arena?"

"In the arena? But how will we catch him?" If I let him go, my charming friend might reveal his bad-boy side in front of all these nice people. In recent weeks he'd been harder and harder to catch in the meadow. When I tried to halter him, Buddy had dodged and galloped away, snorting, rearing, and tearing around the fence line, the mules following him like cardboard characters. When Buddy was fired up, there was no stopping him. One day he'd stolen my hat from my head and carried it off to the other side of the meadow. I'd laughed out loud, though, as he threw it up in the air as if saying, "ha-HA!" and kept on running, only to circle around, pick it up again and fling it like a Frisbee. But Buddy had also nipped me once. That was mostly why'd I'd come to this clinic. When my friend Stephanie told me about Ken helping her with her Friesian gelding Mateo, I'd signed up immediately.

"Oh, don't worry about catching him," Ken says. "He'll be fine. Come and eat."

I take off Buddy's bridle and let him go. Ken shuts the gate as Buddy trots around, then settles into grazing along the edge of the fence.

"How long have you had him?"

"Oh, actually…uh…he's not my horse," I admit, "but I've been spending time with him for about a year now."

How could I recount in a few sentences how Buddy had come into my life? My mother would have said, "Draw the veil!" I was not going to drop the word *cancer* into this bluebird of a day. Instead of explaining, I blurt out something I never expected to say out loud, "But I hope that he might be someday, if my husband and I can afford to buy him." Of course, that day would exist only on a planet where our bank account gushed with fountains of extra cash. But I do not say this to Ken.

After lunch I ask if I should get the bridle.

"Oh, no," Ken says. "Let's just see what he's up to." He grinds his cigarette in the dirt, tosses it into the trash bin, and picks up a dressage whip leaning against the fence. I can't imagine what Ken might do with Buddy without a halter or bridle. But he motions me into the arena and closes the gate. Ken makes a clucking sound and Buddy's head flies up, a piece of grass hanging out of his mouth like a cigarette. When Ken holds out his hand, Buddy takes off in a floating gallop, swinging his head as he whooshes past us, close but just out of reach. My heart flips up a notch. Buddy's tail is straight up like a stick, and it streams out behind him like a flag.

"Now he's being rude," Ken says, without a trace of impatience or anger. "You little shit!" Ken waves his arm at Buddy, who wags his head just a few feet from Ken's shoulder. "You think you're going to bite me, do you?" Buddy feints left, then gallops around again snorting fiercely, nostrils flaring. Ken snaps the three-foot whip against his leg, forcing Buddy to turn in the opposite direction, his mane flying like a white wing, showing us he is king of the sky. But then Buddy spots something moving outside of the arena and he dodges and bolts past Ken.

"He's afraid now, see?" Ken says. Buddy gallops full out. The whites of his eyes are like moons. "He's scared himself; if we're not careful, he'll lose his head." I know that horses are flight animals, and everything that frightens them is connected to prey behavior. The reason horses survived at all—millions of years before humans—was their ability to escape predators. Clearly, Buddy is wired for flight. Ken turns to all of us, "To a horse, every blue tarp in the wind..." (or, I thought, each rattly bucket on their back) "...is a potential death threat, a cougar ready to pounce."

When Buddy gallops back, Ken sends him in the other direction. Buddy tosses his head, blows his nostrils, and sidesteps like a gymnast. But this time, instead of swinging his arm in defense, Ken begins to laugh.

"Wait a minute. This horse is not out to threaten me. Yes, he thinks he's a big shot, and he's a bit of an asshole, but actually—no, he's a clown! Look at him! Everyone laughs as Buddy calms down, prances around nodding his head, showing off like a kid who has run away from his mom but does a cartwheel to charm her anyway.

"This horse is in love with his own body," Ken says, and we all silently agree as Buddy glides by like a dancer.

Ken approaches Buddy again, this time striding toward him, then backing up, just like a dancer himself. He snaps the whip not to hit or scare Buddy, but to get his attention. Buddy comes to a full stop, his tracks making an *11* in the dust.

"It's a lot about pressure," Ken says to me. "Actually, the release of pressure. Horses learn not from the pressure itself, but the absence of it. That's how they talk." He moves toward Buddy, then backs off when Buddy recoils slightly, as if they are one breathing lung. When Ken steps back, Buddy comes toward him cautiously.

"There's an invisible pocket of energy between you and your horse. When you release the energy it's a reward. When you give clear intention with it, it has meaning and power. Horses are always looking for that safety."

Sure enough, as Ken holds out his hand as an invitation, Buddy walks straight toward him, ears forward, curious. Ken allows Buddy to touch his outstretched fingers and then, with a tiny step toward him, he clucks, asking him to step back. Buddy does so immediately and stands open-faced, ready for what's next.

"He's had somebody work him hard in the past," Ken says. "Someone has chased him around. Did you see the way he responded to my tiny pressure before?"

Fred had told me Buddy was saved from an exotic animal farm— where he was confined knee-deep in manure before he ended up with a local woman. And then Fred.

Buddy follows Ken like a puppy. When Ken stops walking, Buddy stops, too. I marvel. No bridle. No halter. Just two guys taking a stroll.

"Catching a horse? Nipping? Problems with the bit? Head tossing? They're all the same, really," Ken tells us. "Once you get right with the horse—when you address the fear, the confusion, or the past—and provide strong, calm leadership, these things will disappear. Buddy reaches over with his nose, and Ken politely clucks at him to keep his distance. Buddy backs up and lets out a big sigh. Spaciousness surrounds all three of us. I feel my own body relax.

Ken turns to me. "Whatever you don't know about yourself, your horse'll show you. If you're impatient, he'll be afraid. If you're not focused and clear, he will reflect your distraction."

Ken wiggles his index finger in the air, and Buddy moves back another step.

"Buddy will be more comfortable and less naughty when you are clear about your own intention. And—by the way…," Ken says, "you are not a scratching post. I saw him with you over there at the gate watching the other lessons."

Ken must have eyes in the back of his head.

"When you rode in this morning, I knew you two were a unit. You clearly have a connection with this horse." I reach out and touch Buddy's neck as if to confirm what Ken is saying. Buddy has a way of making bad things shrink and disappear.

"But when you were standing by the gate earlier? I saw some disrespect. Were you aware of that?" Ken takes the bridle from the fencepost, puts it on Buddy, and rubs his forehead. Buddy blinks, obedient and relaxed. "It isn't good for you or for Buddy to allow him to do that. He needs the solid assurance that you respect yourself."

Ken's words stir something deep inside me. They are true about Buddy, with whom I am deeply smitten, but they also resonate with what had happened years before, when I was blown from one life into another. Which, in turn, had brought me to this very afternoon. Like Buddy, I'd seen my share of wild relationships—both human and animal. And I, too, had lost my head a few times. Maybe that's why I felt such a kinship with this horse. Ken's lesson revealed that Buddy and I were actually afraid of the same things: Death. Entrapment. Being misunderstood. And mistreated, yes. But there was something else.

Ken hands me Buddy's reins and adjusts his hat. "I mean, would you want a person to come up and do that to you? Push you around, invade your space? Would you stand there and take it just because you loved him?"

Chapter 2.

⋘ The Rope Trail ⋙

In New Mexico, death was always sniffing around the edges. I found myself stopping on the highway to scoot—with a folded newspaper—migrating tarantulas safely to the other side. I hovered over injured magpies to keep the cats away, and I breathed deeply to calm the wave of heat and sorrow when I drove past yet another freshly killed dog along the road. Living in the mountains of Northern New Mexico, so close to the jaws of nature, my skin felt peeled back, everything exposed to the light. I'd been seduced anyway—by its dangerous beauty, off-the-grid artists, ancient pueblos, and the powerful rivers and mountains. All hopelessly alluring.

By the time I reached my late thirties, I'd fallen in love a number of times. Not only with compelling men, but also with geographies. I'd been beguiled by rural Vermont, by England, and after that Boston, a city I came to adore. I always seemed to be chasing a mysterious dream that included my *idea* of a place as much as the place itself: the storybook New England villages along the sleepy Connecticut River, the footpath that led from my house southwest of London to where the Magna Carta was signed, the steeple of the Old North Church I could see from my Boston apartment— these were places where "real stuff" had happened, unlike the wet, mossy coast of Washington where I'd grown up. Captain Puget was the only big star of our history books, which barely mentioned the myriad coastal Indian tribes who'd flourished on our shores long before European explorers cruised in.

To the mild consternation of my parents, I also seemed to choose circumstances that included marginal financial stability, yet promised—and delivered—freedom and adventure. As I see it now, I was driven not by what I wanted to *be* so much as how I wanted to *live*. In fact, the settings, both rural and urban, were integral to that dream—as if watching myself live into a story while creating new ones. The French philosopher Pascal said, "Imagination cannot make fools wise, but she can make them happy." New Mexico unwittingly offered me both: boundless happiness and a strong dose of wisdom.

The spring I was 35 I packed up my Ford Festiva, left Boston, and drove with my black-and-white mustachioed cat, Badger, west to Riojos for the summer. I ended up staying seven years. I taught workshops at the Pueblo and repaired houses with a local carpenter, wrote art reviews for a New Mexico magazine, played my flute at a local pub. And I learned to fly-fish.

After years in Britain and on the East Coast, the space of New Mexico felt like a homecoming, and the life I cobbled together was precarious but exhilarating. On the phone my mother would gently ask about the snowstorms. Did I have snow tires? And how was my bank account? Was Badger managing to dodge the coyotes and the lightning? What about men?

I hadn't a clue, of course, that I would eventually be flushed from that magical place, but in the meantime, I drank up the high desert for all it was worth. I practiced my fly-cast on the Rio Hondo, which flowed right outside my door, and I snagged trout for dinner. Once, after riding a friend's quarter horse gelding far across the mesa, I called my mother just to say, "Mom, I can die now!" And we laughed, she knowing exactly what I meant—that I was so full with my joy, I couldn't imagine more.

When you look back at chapters of your life, though, there are certain moments that stand out as prescient, symbolic. It isn't till later, when you've risen above the chaos, that you see a larger symmetry unfolding. Even now, long after leaving that ravishing sky, I return to a September day I went fishing with my friend Juan. The aspens stippled gold across the Sangre de Christos, and the sky was a deep, cerulean blue. Juan, a novelist, was at least a decade older, an experienced fisherman, and it was always an honor to fish with him.

That afternoon we drove several miles out to the very edge of the vast canyon. He said he wanted to show me the Rope Trail, named for its near-vertical drop from the mesa to the gushing Rio Grande below. The path, hidden from the casual observer, isn't far from the bridge that spans the Gorge. When you drive across the mesa, the bridge—a dizzying 650 feet above the white water—is only visible right before you cross. In an instant the Earth falls away and you are flying over the canyon, its sheer rock cliffs plummeting to the river carving through the fissure. A river guide friend had told me about a cougar who'd attempted to cross that bridge one night. When the cat got to the middle of the trestle, an oncoming car blinded him so completely that in one clean leap, he cleared the guardrail, headlights catching only his disappearing tail. My friend had found the body not far from where Juan and I were headed.

"This way!" Juan hollered as I slammed the truck door. We slipped and skidded down the rocky trail, Juan's red bandana fluttering; I followed his lead. As we descended around giant boulders, he pointed out a red-tail hawk nest tucked in the crevices, white dung splattered over the rocks like Anasazi petroglyphs. Bones of small mammals lay scattered around the nest. The merciless sun glared, and I was careful to keep from pitching downward toward the river below.

Juan scrambled on, pointing to the ravens circling above us on a thermal, their guttural cries echoing off the canyon walls. As we descended, sending a flush of pebbles ahead, we hung to scrub pine and sagebrush, clutching our rod cases, sometimes using them as walking sticks to break a possible fall. When we reached the bottom, the cool river air soothed our faces. We sat on a big rock, put up our rods, and tied on some flies. I played it safe and pulled out a wooly bugger, but Juan tied a complicated double-drop with a nymph on one tippet and an elk-hair caddis on the other.

We began our ritual of leapfrogging. He fished a section, I fished a section, and then when one of us finished, we veered around the other. We worked our way upstream toward the arc of the bridge above us. In my first years of fly-fishing, I'd dreamed about it almost nightly. The smell of cottonwoods on the bank, the perfect cast, and the tug of a trout on the line. I dreamed of rivers I'd never seen and the flow of water moving against my legs. I also had nightmares of landing other creatures: bright green birds with hooks in their beaks or a horse that couldn't untangle itself from the line. Sometimes in my dream I'd start reeling in a submerged beast, and, just when it was about to surface, I'd wake with a jerk, my heart flapping. But mostly I dreamed I was pregnant, filled with a fish growing inside me, moving to the sound of water, the river carrying us faster and faster downstream.

It was strange how fishing awakened the desire for my own spawning. The men I'd been involved with in Riojos had not worked out, however. One had died swiftly and unexpectedly from lung cancer; the other was no longer able to have children. I'd been hopeful for each of those romances. The shock, grief, and disappointment just drove me more deeply to the rivers—the fragrance of cottonwoods, the sound of water over stone. And each time I cast my fly into the current, I think I was also casting for a lasting mate.

The life-giving force of fishing, however, seemed paradoxical to that moment when a trout flupps on the line. After all, predator behavior was new to me. As I'd learned to fish, I also learned that each delicate flip of the line tied me closer to an ancient survival ritual. And each time I felt the rush of a trout on the line and the smatter in the water, I was startled by the unfamiliar elation washing through my body, as though there were something necessary about the swift violence, the death.

Juan and I fished upstream, leapfrogging toward the bridge, its trusses arching high above us like flying buttresses. I cast out over the riffles, and soon I felt that thrilling bump on the line. A silver shower scattered the air as the trout fought and splashed. I set the hook and landed him near the bank.

I blessed the fish over and over again, trying not to drop him in the sand. I blessed him partly to calm myself, partly because I was still not accustomed to the glittery package of life when I finally received it. I breathed in and out, mouthing a grace, smacked its head against a rock, and gently laid it on the fresh grass in my creel, a practice I'd learned from a friend at the Pueblo. I stood up, trembly and dazed, as if I'd just made love.

I tied on a hopper and slowly cast upstream. Just as a cutthroat rose to my fly, a sound like dynamite exploded in the middle of the river. I drew back as the bursting *PLASHT* echoed off the canyon walls. In a split second Juan yelled, "Ruuuuuuuuun!" and then "Cover your head!" My animal instincts were already moving my body toward the shadow of the bridge. I followed Juan as fast as I could over the slippery rocks, the fly on my line looping in the air like penmanship.

"There's kids up there! Damn them!" Juan, said, out of breath. He squinted skyward. Sure enough, we could just make out the heads of two teenage boys leaning over the railing hundreds of feet above us. One of them held another huge stone over his head. When the boy let go of the small boulder it seemed to take forever to fall, like a slow-motion clip in a movie. I tried to calculate where it would land but followed Juan's lead and froze. It finally crashed with a huge commotion just a short cast from where we stood, water rising in a violent plume. My hands shook, as if we were being hunted. Nowhere to hide. It was useless to yell over the roar of the river, so we warily watched the boys until they finally ambled to the other side of the bridge then disappeared.

We'd lost our enthusiasm, and there was nothing to do but head home. In any other place one might have reported those kids to the police, but such occurrences were common in Northern New Mexico, like lightning on the mesa, bubonic plague rampant in the prairie dogs, flash floods down the arroyos, loose horses struck by drunk drivers, or the domestic murders that never got solved. The longer I lived there, the more I was privy to the whisper of death always lurking below the surface.

I often think about that day in the Gorge—a slippery descent into a deep canyon, dodging more and more stones, and the long, slow ascent back to high ground. But that day I wasn't dwelling on darkness; I was too busy falling in love with the glittery trout wrapped in grass in my creel, the fading light washing the Pueblo's sacred mountain a deep lavender, and the thrill of having survived falling rocks. When we emerged onto the mesa, Juan and I laughed at what we'd eluded and popped open a couple of beers from his cooler. He said he couldn't wait to tell his girlfriend. The only thing missing in my life, I thought, as the old truck bumped across the mesa toward town, was a good man. After five years in this intoxicating place, I needed someone with whom I could share this sky, someone to "ride the river with," as my fly-fisherman grandfather used to say. It was no coincidence that the New Mexico state license plate was emblazoned with "Land of Enchantment."

Chapter 3.

⋙ *The Beltane Fires* ⋘

WITHIN A WEEK AFTER THAT day with Juan, a painter friend asked if I'd like to meet his pal visiting from Chicago—apparently a world-class fly-fisherman—looking for angling companions in the area. "You guys have a lot in common," Pasco said. "Would you be willing to share a secret fishing spot or two? I think you'll like him. I knew his father back in the day, and I've known Trey for years." The following Saturday I was hiking another trail to the Rio Grande, several miles downstream from the Rope Trail. This one, however, was not steep and did not include a bridge where stones could fly. It was one of my favorite places to fish; I loved the way that big river shouldered through the Gorge, a hidden pool at every bend.

Trey was a paragon of enthusiasm. We'd been talking nonstop since he'd picked me up in his red Trooper, and we arrived at the trailhead in high spirits. Tall, affable, with jet-black hair, his mind was agile and curious. Not to mention his accent. He told me he'd grown up in the Scottish Highlands. "The lochs and streams taught me the language of trout!" he said with a tongue-in-cheek flourish, grinning at me briefly while tying a double-hackle onto his tippet. His smile was generous, and his long fingers tied the knot with ease.

I learned he was a dealer of antiquarian books, mostly natural history. Birds in particular, but birds of prey were his specialty, he said. He'd come west to Santa Fe to appraise the library of a collector who'd recently died. "It's a big collection and it's going to take some time, but I'm hoping to find some hidden treasures." He bit off the extra line with his front teeth. Trey had been married, he told me, had three children, eventually divorced, and left Britain for America. He'd been living in Chicago ever since.

"Fishing has always kept me out of trouble," he smiled, and I smiled back. His eyes were clear and green as water. Standing there in his seasoned fishing vest and waders, his long limbs emanated a familiarity with pleasure and appetite. He wore an aristocratic air. Pasco's instincts were right. In less than an hour, Trey and I had entered a space that cast most everything else in a drab light. When he told me he'd be in Santa Fe for at least a month, I was already thinking about a couple of streams north of Riojos. I suppose I was sending out pheromones, or maybe we both were. Looking back at it now, my brain was not a major player in his gravitational pull. My body was thinking for me.

Trey closed his fly box with a click and slipped it into his vest pocket. I vaguely compared his tidy system to my confusion of flies stuffed into an Altoids tin. While we walked downstream toward some good riffles we discovered yet another connection: we'd both grown up with horses. While I'd just had one horse, his father had had a string of hunters and thoroughbreds. "Dad insisted that my sister and I know how to jump, especially riding to hounds." (*Riding to hounds!*) I pictured him as a child galloping over fences in the Highlands when I was galloping Lightfoot bareback along the tide flats of Puget Sound. He told me that his dad would yell at him when he fell off, and he'd disappear into the glen with the falcons he'd raised.

"Falcons? You mean like hawks?"

"Yes, I raised them for years. For hunting grouse. My dad wasn't ever interested in them. He was too busy with his work. I learned about hawking from a local man. It was just what I needed. Of course, I had them when I was married with kids, too. But I'd never have a hawk again." We waded into the big river.

"Why not?" I'd never met a falconer before.

"Too addictive. Too obsessive," he said, laughing. "I gave it up when I left Britain five years ago." Trey waved his hand toward the river and beyond, as if it were a Celtic landscape. "I loved all the freedom as a child, though. It was how I survived, really. My mum—she was Italian—died when I was a teenager. And my dad was gone a lot." A deep sadness flickered over his forehead, then disappeared. I learned that his father, a well-known artist, had died, ten years before. I remembered reading his obituary when I lived in London; I'd seen his paintings there as well as several shows in America. This added an extra zing to my already-electric attraction to this man.

Within the first or second cast, Trey had a big rainbow on. It flapped wildly as the line went taut, then skidded across the riffles. In a flash of silver, it had dipped under the surface, revealing a glinting fin, then thrashed against the current and the inevitable tug of the hook. Trey expertly removed the fly, then held the trout under the water so it faced upstream to orient itself. "Go," he said. "Get on with you." The trout hung in a kind of daze and finally shot out into the current.

Trey caught and released several fish that afternoon, and I landed one. I admired how efficient he was in claiming his catch. Our lexicons were stocked with so many of the same words: Creel and cinch. Tippet and tack. Rod and rein. Words that conjure whole worlds. Even the fly Trey chose that day was a promising sign. The double-hackle had been my grandfather Boppa's favorite.

Before throwing my gear into the back seat of Trey's Trooper, I snapped a small branch of sagebrush, pinched it, and inhaled its fragrance. In New Mexico I never knew what would happen next. One day I'm eating scrambled eggs alone with my cats, and the next I'm fly-fishing with someone who just about fits my perfect-man template.

When Trey pulled out onto the highway, our rod cases rolled around together in the back seat and landed on top of each other. His canvas case had well-worn leather handles, the kind you might see in an old anglers' catalog alongside split-willow creels. The tag was also evocative: in neat, handwritten script was an address in Inverness. He turned to me and smiled, "At least we know our fly rods are compatible!" We held a mutual grin for an extra beat. He turned his attention back to the road. "Fancy some dinner before I head back to Santa Fe?"

Within days Trey had called to invite me on a fishing trip with Pasco. They'd be coming through Riojos, he said, on their way to Jicarilla Apache land for the weekend. Why didn't I come along? The early May day was bright but chilly, and there were still patches of snow on the pass. When Pasco's truck finally bumped over the potholes to a campsite right by the lake, we weren't surprised the place was empty. Even the willows still held their buds closed. A thin wind blew across the water, making ripples like folds in a Navajo blanket.

Pasco set up his three-man tent and another tent for gear while Trey and I laid a fire for later. They'd each brought small, inflatable float tubes and flippers. I'd borrowed a rubber raft with oars. While they bobbed around in the calm inlet, my raft was blown all the way across the lake. From a distance I could see Trey casting in easy arcs, his torso emerging from the deep. Except for the ratchety sound of reels and a raven heading home, it was quiet and strangely desolate. Soon a full and ready moon rose over the rock cliffs and lit the whole lake like a mirror.

I paddled back to shore with two fish and arrived at a blazing campfire. Pasco brought out a dish of cannelloni he'd made beforehand and heated it up in the fire. We drank wine and watched the flames lick the air. Trey sat next to me, and when his elbow touched mine, a zipper-like rush coursed through my limbs. The flames grew taller, casting shadows against the pines behind our campsite.

"Hey, it's the first of May," Trey said. "Beltane Fires."

"What the hell is Beltane Fires?" Pasco took another swig of red wine.

Trey zipped up his down jacket. "An ancient Celtic ritual. Every year at this time, I guess the tribes lit these wild, smashing bonfires and shed their clothes."

"Sounds good so far," Pasco said.

"Yes, well it gets better. Apparently, they all sort of let loose in a kind of manic, one-night mating-fest, planting (along with their crops) as many seeds as possible. Quite a rumpus!" Pasco and I cracked up, mostly at Trey's choice of words.

Trey said, "The only problem I can figure is that they must have frozen their bums off. May 1st in Italy is one thing, but in Britain?!" We pictured a clan of naked druids prancing (and shivering) in the chilly northern night. No danger of such a spectacle here. We all moved nearer to the fire as the wind picked up.

The three of us bedded down in Pasco's large tent, three sleeping bags, foot-to-head—me on the end. Coyotes howled in a circle just beyond our campsite. Then came another sound, a weird *smack* and then a splash. It sounded like someone was firing a gun, but when Pasco pulled back the tent flap there was nothing there. The smashing got louder, though. "I'm going out to see what's going on—" Pasco pulled on his boots and disappeared into the milky night. Trey and I lay breathless, only the goose down of our sleeping bags between us.

"It's a beaver for Chrissake," Pasco said, crawling back inside. "Slapping his tail against the water like a maniac."

"He's wooing the woman of his dreams, Pasco," Trey said.

"I'm going to sleep in the gear tent," Pasco said, dragging his sleeping bag out the flap. "Maybe I'll get more shut-eye farther away from the lake and that damned beaver. He doesn't sound like he's stopping anytime soon."

"Give him credit, Pasco," Trey said as the tent flap closed. "He's fired up by the Beltane Fires." Pasco grumbled, and soon his snoring reached us all the way from the far tent. Within moments my head and Trey's head were no longer at each other's feet. Not a goose feather between us.

Chapter 4.

⤳ *Softness* ⤳

BUDDY PRANCES AROUND ME WHILE I stand tall, holding tight to the reins. His neck is arched, his ears pricked. He looks like a brave and noble desert horse. I secretly love it when he gets ramped up and snorty; I think it's a tribute to my horsemanship that I can handle a hot-blooded horse, not only from the ground but riding, as well.

Ken thinks otherwise. "Don't be seduced by the bling," he says, turning to me. "Yes, he's handsome, but he's not listening to you at all."

"His ears are forward." I admire Buddy's shapely head. "Look! He's cheery." Buddy's elegant lines remind me of those swooshy sumi paintings I'd done in junior high when my father had brought me ink and brushes from a business trip to Japan.

"Oh, he's not necessarily cheery. He's just checking out that dog over there in the field." Ken points. I look behind me, and sure enough, Buddy has spotted a black Lab snuffling around in the weeds.

Ken takes a drag on his cigarette, holds it for several seconds then exhales, blowing the smoke over his left shoulder. This is my second time at the Fairgrounds with Ken, and I had counted the days to get here this late September Saturday. After the first lesson, it was if someone had given me the taste of an exotic drug; I wanted more. Buddy and I had arrived that morning before anyone else, and this time I'd brought my notebook, a pen, and a crumpled list of questions for Ken.

I am still puzzled about the time, not long after I'd met Buddy, when he had reached over and bitten me on the forearm. He'd drawn blood. I'd gone home, washed the wound with rubbing alcohol, and wept. I took it all personally, the dream of my new healing-horse-friend shattered. In the year since, I'd gotten over it (and he had never done it again), but I was still troubled by Buddy's occasional bad behavior.

With great apprehension I tell Ken about the nipping, and he just waves his hand. "When Buddy is confident with you as a partner, that will be a nonissue. It just won't happen." He takes the reins from me as he had done the last time and backs Buddy up. When Buddy resists and drags his feet like a recalcitrant child, Ken stands up tall and gently snaps the dressage whip on the ground. Buddy, like radar, beams all his attention on Ken, as if saying, "Oh. Gee!! Okay. What do I do now?" When Ken lifts an eyebrow, Buddy backs two more steps.

I always wondered how Buddy could scatter the mules from his hay pile with a mere glance. Gracie would squeak and Molly listed to the left if Buddy so much as wiggled an ear. In all my years with Lightfoot, or even the horses I'd ridden in England and New Mexico, I had not consciously thought about this thing Ken was showing me.

"It's called softness," Ken says, asking Buddy to give way gently as he steps toward him. He goes on to describe the invisible elasticity in the horse's body. "It's a place of balance and unity in the horse's movement as well as a harmony between you and the horse." Buddy relaxes when Ken turns toward me. "We look for it on the ground and when we're in the saddle." I'd had a glimmer of feeling this with Lightfoot. I remembered the lightness in the mouth, the easy flow of motion. I knew his every move in those first years when he followed me everywhere and came when I called. Often, I'd ride him up to the stable without a saddle or bridle. But as I got older and indoctrinated into lead changes, figure eights, equitation classes, and 4-H horse-show ribbons, it became more about getting and doing rather than actually listening and being.

Some other kids' horses behaved with a kind of liquid grace, but often they'd been "professionally trained," a mysterious term used for horses that belonged to kids whose parents had a lot of dough. But Ken was making it clear that "professionally trained" did not always mean a happy horse—or even a dependable one. I thought of that Morgan mare in the last lesson.

"Most times, these poor horses look good in the show ring," Ken draws the last out of his cigarette, "but they are pulled, braced, and contorted into the things they are made to do. Instead of offering free and balanced carriage, they are pulled into what is often called a 'frame.'"

"What we ultimately want," Ken reaches out his hand, asking Buddy to touch it, "is to offer our horses a choice. We want to make it easy for them. If I show Buddy how unstressful it is to stand quietly with me," he drops his hand and Buddy relaxes, "then he will actually want to be with me instead of being forced to and resenting it." Buddy's long pink tongue emerges from his licorice lips. Even his tongue delights me, and I laugh and touch his neck. A couple of the horses outside the arena blow their nostrils in a release of their own breath.

"See?" Ken says. "We're getting our lick and chew now. When a horse licks and chews, he is releasing tension." Ken adjusts his hat and stands up a little straighter. "He is present, and he's actually digesting what has just taken place, letting go of the tension." I, too, feel calm and safe, noticing my own breathing has changed.

"It's important we let him have that time to process." Buddy yawns and he no longer resembles that fired-up boy who'd been prancing around me earlier. I loved that part of a horse—the wild part I could "handle"—but I can see what Ken is talking about. Buddy is relaxed, not ramped up and distracted.

"This may not be your *fantasy* of being with Buddy," Ken waves his arm in a big arc, "galloping on a white horse with orchestral music playing in the background." We laugh. "But I promise you: Reality is better than the dream."

Buddy's ears swivel when Ken zips up his jacket against the wind. "It's more honest this way," he says. "More comfortable for the horse. See?" He nods toward Buddy, whose eyes are soft. "He's with us now, part of the family—the herd. Not off with that dog in the field."

Chapter 5.

Home Ranch

RIGHT BEFORE TREY WHOOSHED INTO my life, I'd moved with Badger and a new cat, Callie, to an old compound called the Rocking H Ranch. The pink adobe structures looked as though they'd risen right out of the earth. Built in the 1930s by a landscape painter who'd run a string of horses for Hollywood movies, apparently the ranch had been a magnet for many artist parties. I pictured the pink bathtub in my casita filled to the brim with champagne bottles on ice. And, though it was no longer a working ranch, you could almost see the ponies kicking up dust. The best part was I lived right next door to my artist friend Sas.

In addition to the four or five dwellings, the Ranch had an old pump house, a vegetable garden, a huge locust tree in the courtyard, and a view of the Picuris Range to the south. So when Trey's Santa Fe sublet ended, he moved in with me—six weeks after the Beltane Fires—and the Ranch took on a whole new life. Trey went gangbusters with the garden, helping Sas plant vegetables, and, by midsummer, the huge plot was overflowing. "Our Eden!" Trey would say, proudly bringing in squash and broccoli rabe for me to cook for dinner. After a day of work, often Sas and I sat on her patio drinking Campari and soda while the sun set over the Picuris. "Sublime," she would say, as the wind rustled in the giant locust tree. And then again, "Sublime."

When another space came up for rent, I'd urged Trey to nab it since it was getting pretty tight in my small space. (Trey alone seemed to occupy whole rooms and more.) This way at least we both could work in peace. And peaceful it was. Trey focused on his book business, Sas was busy with a new series of painted assemblages, and I was teaching at the Pueblo. Each morning Trey and I sipped coffee under the locust tree, laughing at the magpies holding forth in the branches above, Trey reading from *Fathers and Sons* by Turgenev or *The Compleat Angler* by Izaak Walton. At night Trey and I would disappear into his casita and slip into his king-sized bed, the stone fountain outside his window burbling in the night.

By August we were off on another fishing trip, this time to the Nevada-Oregon border, where friends of Trey's owned a working cattle ranch. Afterward we planned to head north to Washington State so he could meet my family. Trey's red Trooper was packed to the gills with maps, fishing books, novels, bird books, and brand-new camping gear he'd bought (proudly) himself.

"The Florys are super people," Trey said, "Salt of the earth. Welcoming as can be. You'll love them. Three brothers, three families, one ranch. Just like *Bonanza*! There's something about the way they live…It's just that—they make a real living, you know? They're not pretend." Trey had told me about his own sister, a lead singer for an R&B band, and his half-sister, a model. Even with his father dead, his family was tough to compete with, and talking about them often made him anxious. Apparently, they didn't get along well, and he barely mentioned the years he'd tried to become a painter like his dad. His father had sent him to the top art school in Britain, but Trey had not thrived there, and his father finally cut off his tuition, telling him to "go be the President of Wales or something." Trey turned inward to books and had found solace in reading everything from philosophy and poetry to political and natural history. By doing so, he also fulfilled his own thwarted visual aesthetic, collecting volumes that were physical works of art themselves.

I didn't care that he wasn't outwardly successful like his family. In fact, I admired how he had chosen what I saw as a richer path. Instead of celebrity, he'd retreated to nature. Instead of moneygrubbing, he made a living (small though it was) from another kind of art. Plus, his life was chock-full of intriguing people, and he was game to take off at a moment's notice. Our kinship grew into a fusion of high spirits; we knew what each other was going to say before we said it. That summer Trey introduced me to the work of Buddhist teacher Pema Chodron, and we lapped up her writing and listened to her CD series about the practice of lovingkindness. Trey laughed about his lack of worldly riches, "but I have a *wealth* of knowledge!" he said, holding me close in bed. We could talk all night. In fact, we did. Often we were "knackered" (Trey's word) in the morning because we didn't want to waste our time sleeping when there was so much to say, so much to find out about each other and the world. When we did finally sleep, we'd sometimes awaken to discover we'd actually dreamed the same dream.

This western road trip appealed to both our imaginations. Trey's long fingers gripped the steering wheel as he pointed the Trooper across the high desert. I loved his hands, their lightness and how they held a fly rod. In the short time we'd been together their touch had already given me pleasure beyond my imagination. And now we were headed to a blue-ribbon trout stream *and* cattle to wrangle by horseback. Not to mention the mythic Florys.

We sped past red rock cliffs and wide mesas spotted with sage. "The gods conspired to bring us together, don't you think?" Trey looked over at me. I agreed and rolled down the window, the dry air filling the car. "And I truly think the American West is my true home. The expanse of it! Who knew it could go on and on like this?"

Trey adjusted his wire-framed glasses, then reached over to squeeze my hand. "And darling, aren't you glad we're grown-ups?" I didn't know exactly what he meant and hadn't really thought about grown-upness in light of our love affair—after all I was in my late thirties and he was seven years older. But his comment implied that we had "arrived." From somewhere. Together. I loved the together part. The fusion I had with Trey was completely new to me. I had never surrendered so completely to another person. Physically, psychically.

I stuck my arm out to feel the breeze. A Cooper's hawk caught a thermal, and Trey pointed out that it had spotted a rodent. The bird spiraled, then dropped to the ground in a swoop. I imagined the small deer mouse in the shadow of that hawk right before the end. Trey clutched the wheel and rocked gently back and forth as he drove, smiling with joy. The desert unrolled before us like a storyline.

That night we stopped for an early supper, then drove up into the mountains, veering off on a logging road to look for a place to car-camp. After a day of constant chatter, we got quiet as the light faded and finally decided on a grassy spot just off the dirt road. In the dark, I pulled out the sleeping gear while Trey began to set up the tent. Soon I heard soft cursing inside our half-erected love nest.

"Can I help?" I peered in, ready to offer some quip about assemblage.

I switched on my flashlight to reveal his face contorted with frustration. His hands were shaking, bending the tent pole so hard it looked like it was going to break. Then he clumsily jammed the pole through the fabric hem. It got stuck and he threw it on the ground. "Bloody hell. Just leave me be." His voice wasn't familiar, its timbre unnerving.

"There's no need to get upset, Trey," I said, trying to sound sooth-ing. "We've had such a happy day. Let's not let a simple tent ruin it." It occurred to me that he might not be experienced in camping—or with tents. He'd been telling me about the lodges he'd stayed in when he'd gone hawking and fishing in Britain. And, except for the fire, Pasco had set up camp on our fishing trip. I squatted next to him, thinking of my dad saying, "Spilt milk? Broken cups? We don't let these things bother us!" But Trey was clearly bothered; all his energy was focused on that tent pole, as if it would bring him down if he didn't fight it. An owl hooted in the trees, and some-where a bird was disturbed from its night's sleep.

After a tense moment, I wondered if he was going to break the pole on purpose. I'd had other boyfriends who occasionally lashed out at recalcitrant objects. But Trey finally dropped it, the canvas sagging from its clumsy curve. "I'm sorry," he said. "I just can't help myself sometimes." The spell was broken, and I picked up the other end of the pole. I caught a glimmer of a little boy caught in a web of fear and inadequacy. Clearly his dad didn't have my dad's view of spilt milk. I slowly threaded the tent pole through the canvas pocket, and soon we managed to settle down. It felt like a victory that we'd worked this out. Together. We fell into a deep slumber.

In the morning when I woke, Trey was stroking my head and kissing my ear. I knew it was his way of thanking me for getting him through the previous night's hiccup. He made love to me fiercely in the dappled sunlight. Chickadees chirped in the trees. We packed up the Trooper and headed west, leaving behind the memory of that silly tent.

The Florys' Oregon Ranch sprawled for hundreds of acres across a valley snugged up to Bureau of Land Management land. When we arrived, Trey and I were already slated to accompany the youngest of the three Flory brothers to fetch some cattle in the hills the next day. Trey grinned and put his arm around my shoulders, knowing just how happy this would make me. I melted into his side. He was right about my delight, and not only that, he was slowly becoming my Nathan Sinclair.

As a teenager, I'd fantasized about Nathan Sinclair, the name I gave my imaginary boyfriend: A tall cowboy gifted with horses who also read books, discussed ideas, and knew about art. He lived on a ranch surrounded by cottonwood trees next to a mountain stream somewhere in Montana or one of the big western states. Except for the cowboy part, Trey was beginning to fill his shoes. I say shoes, because Trey didn't own cowboy boots, but before the trip I'd helped him buy a pair in Santa Fe.

When I was twelve, my mother gave me all her precious novels by the cowboy writer Will James, whose distinctive line drawings accompanied his stories of the American West. I read *All in the Day's Riding, Horses I've Known, Big-Enough,* and *Home Ranch,* convinced I was born in the wrong decade and the wrong part of the country. Deep into those Will James stories I breathed cotton-woods along a river, sagebrush, and the dusty trails; I could feel the snow against my face. I learned new words for landscape like *wash* and *draw,* words for cattle dealers like *outfit,* and clothing terms, too, especially *chaps*—pronounced "shaps." I not only admired, I *was* that cowboy riding through the sagebrush.

I often pictured myself in a world far from the wet, dark nights of the Washington coast. I sat by a campfire on a high mesa, my bedroll stretched out under the spiky stars. In seventh grade study hall, when I was supposed to be doing algebra, I sneaked a chapter or two from *The Drifting Cowboy* or *Sand,* and then I'd make my own pencil drawings of horses, trying to catch the curve of the neck, the arched tail.

When Billy Flory showed us our horses the next morning, I had to pinch myself; the Flory ranch was Will James and Nathan

Sinclair rolled into one. At 6:00 a.m. we'd eaten at the bunkhouse with the ranch hands, then led our horses to the barn to saddle up. Trey looked so handsome on his roan mare. He had a good seat, even if he was a little tight with the reins. I mounted Ribbon, my paint gelding, and loped ahead with Trey to catch up with the cowhands. Our orders were to find some stray calves up in the hills among the scrub pine and in some hidden canyons. I liked the way my horse used his haunches to propel himself forward, then turn easily with a slight shift of my weight. I urged him toward the trail, following a hand named Pete on a sorrel. "We're headed up there," Pete said, pointing out a cut in the sagebrush-covered hills. Trey trotted beside me and we lined out. The hands gave us a lot of room for error that day, but we cheered when we managed to bring the missing calves home. A red-tailed hawk circled in the gyre above us. I couldn't wait to tell my mother everything.

The next night at the ranch house barbeque, Billy Flory recited his cowboy poetry, and we all applauded and had more watermelon. Afterward Trey and I put up our fly rods and meandered down to the river. We fished till dusk, the evening hatch hovering above the river, luring trout to the surface, one of those nights when every cast seems magical. Each time you think it's your last, you can't leave the pucker on the pools, fish kissing the surface for a fly. We caught enough trout for breakfast and released the rest. We were just ready to walk back to the cabin before it got too dark, when Trey said, "Whoa!!" A black object swung from his line, back and forth across the surface of the water. Trey reeled it in as it fluttered through the air.

"It's a bat!" he said. "I've caught a bat." Sure enough, the tiny creature had dived for Trey's swirling fly and snagged its poor webby wing on the hook.

"Oh, no!" I cried.

"Get a cloth or something! Quick," Trey said, and I raced up to the cabin and brought back a bath towel. Trey had lowered the leathery fellow to the riverbank. The human-like fear on its tiny face was a mirror of my own. His eyes met mine, and his baby fingers tried to grab the edge of the towel. Trey managed to cover up every part of the bat's body but the pierced wing. We leaned over, holding our breath as Trey carefully pulled out the hook.

"Voilà!" Trey held up the elk-hair caddis. No blood came from the wound, so we lifted the cloth. The trembling creature shook for a moment, then looked skyward. In an instant he was airborne, and in three or four loops disappeared into the thickening darkness. I slid my arm around Trey's waist, leaned my head against his shoulder, and we sat in silence while the river gushed by, the night wrapping its soft blanket around us.

When we went back, we fell immediately into bed, the smell of cottonwoods wafting through our private cabin. We talked about the tiny bat and how vulnerable it had seemed. And we recalled Billy's poems, how everyone had loved them. Because Trey was such a voracious reader, and a good listener, I reluctantly confessed to him my doubts about my own poetry—if I was good enough. He held me tighter, "Oh, every serious artist feels this way, my love, that they don't measure up. Or that they're a fraud. But isn't your worry actually proof of your devotion? How truly married you are to the work? And if it makes a difference, I think your poems are splendid. Beautiful and splendid. Just like you."

I kissed his smooth shoulder, then lay back and blinked at the dark ceiling, wondering how I'd found someone who knew me in ways I didn't understand myself; it felt like I'd come home.

Then Trey began to imagine our future child. I'd never allowed myself to fantasize about children so recklessly, but Trey was insistent. "You do want a child, don't you? I mean, you're pushing 40. You need a child."

"Well, yes," I said cautiously, my blood growing hot just thinking about it. Our lovemaking was always passionate, tender, and magical, as if we had been planning something larger than "us" all along.

"Well, I can give you one!" He laid his hand on my belly. "Let's let the gods have their way."

Of course I wanted a baby. How could I *not* want to be a parent if, for as long as I remembered, my mother had hugged me and said, "*How* could I be so lucky as to have *you?*" I know she felt the same about my older brother, Paul, and my younger sister, Rosemary—all of us born four years apart.

Motherhood seemed like second nature to me. Even Mom told me once, "Oh, being a mother is like taking care of kittens and dogs and hens and horses, but even better." The big hitch was that my life had never seemed to accommodate children. Most of the men I'd been involved with had been as unprepared as I was to provide a stable place for a child. Even marriage, itself a huge consideration, seemed to be for people with life insurance, jobs, and cars that didn't break down.

After years of preventing pregnancy, though, I was suddenly welcoming the possibility. This seems wildly reckless now—I'd only known this man a few months, and I hadn't a clue what was involved with raising a child. I only knew it seemed good, and right, bountiful and timely. My body was saying *yesyesyesyes* to a biological imperative beyond reason or even my control. It was intoxicating. Once a couple years before Trey, I'd told Mom that it looked like I might never have kids. "Well," she said, "if you have children, you know…you'll never be *free*. You will always be torn." I'd let the silence fill the phone line. She'd never said a thing like that before. I could picture her sweeping her hand out toward the sky. "Children are never really 'gone' even if they've moved away. You worry. You always hope that they are happy. And safe."

It was the first time I really understood that my mother still worried about me and my siblings. Of course having a grown-up child had not entered my storyline. So far, I was intent on the baby part. But I did wonder how Trey and I could afford a child. He survived on a meager inheritance from his father, along with his antique book sales. I wasn't sure how dependable that was. "I'm unemployable!" Trey often said proudly.

"Let's make a child," he said.

"What will we name him?" I asked. Trey licked my ear.

"Why, Zeus, of course!" He rolled over and nearly crushed me.

He smelled like sex and river and dust.

Chapter 6.

False Join-Up

IN KEN'S HORSEMANSHIP, THE TERM for when a horse chooses human company is *join-up*. It's when the horse decides to come to you at liberty—free of saddle, bridle, or halter—instead of choosing its own kind or the wild (even if the wild is only the far end of a corral). Some horsemen call this "hooked on," "being with you," or even "to feel of it," but it's all about the horse finding safety and comfort with a person, without the incentive of a carrot or shaking a bucket of grain. Like Ken, many horsemen and women prefer to work their horses in a large rectangular arena. The Spanish trainers like a smaller square space called a *picadero*. Cowboys prefer a round pen, forty to sixty feet in diameter, to keep a horse moving, so it can't hide in the corners.

After seeing Ken in action, I am excited to try my first attempt at "join-up," and the Fairgrounds round pen—right near the arena—is the perfect spot. Though I'd worked with Ken only a few times, I'd also been watching other clinicians' training videos online. I even ordered a "carrot stick," a tool named and made famous by one of the popular couples of the "natural horsemanship" training movement. The stick is really just a crude form of a dressage whip that directs a horse and never strikes him as punishment. I am so ready to try this "join-up" thing with Buddy, I can taste it. A friend comes along to take a cell phone video.

Unlike many Arabian horses these days, which are often over-bred for long, skinny necks and exaggerated dished faces, Buddy's confirmation reflects an older type of that breed, the kind my grandfather bred: smaller, but more robust, with stouter proportions. Mom told us Boppa's Arab stallion, Miras, was his pride and joy. She loved describing their farm and the beautiful mares who carried Miras's foals. Her father was as exacting and careful with his horses, she said, as he was about fly-fishing. By the time I was old enough to hear these stories, Boppa and my grandmother had sold the farm, but when horses came up in conversation, he got a wistful, faraway look in his eye.

Today in his fuzzy winter coat, Buddy looks more like a yak from the Mongolian Steppes than the Arabian Desert. He prances and dances as I lead him into the round pen. When I go to the center of the ring and turn him loose, he puffs, huffs, and dashes away from me. His tail shoots up, and he begins to gallop too fast for the small space. It is exactly what he'd done at first with Ken that day in the bigger arena, but I don't have Ken's skill, nor does this space seem big enough to contain him. When Buddy rockets around and around, his eyes wild, nostrils snorting, I know things are out of control. The more confined he feels, the more hyped-up he becomes.

All I see in my mind's eye is his leg catching in the fence. Finally, the fear is too much for me, and I turn away, praying out loud that he'll stop. He immediately puts on the brakes and steps toward the center of the pen. I can't believe it. I reach out my hand and Buddy comes in slowly—snorting. Then he begins to follow me around. Anywhere I go Buddy is right with me, his head in line with my shoulder. I am thrilled, as if a runaway lover has fallen back in love with me again. I'm not sure what I've done, but whatever it is, it is working. And it's documented on video!

I immediately email the video to Ken, proud of what I'd experienced my first time alone with Buddy at liberty. I watch the short clip over and over again on my computer, dominated by the image of me in my huge down coat grinning like a lovesick girl, Buddy in his own winter coat mincing his steps toward me.

"Hate to disappoint you," Ken says on the phone. "But that's a false join-up."

"What?" I say, my heart sinking. I'd not heard that term, but I did remember that a friend who'd attended a California trainers' clinic had said that his "join-up" idea was merely a gimmick, nothing about connection or relationship. It had no meaning with the horses; he just frightened them so they sought the only quiet place they could find—in the center with the human.

"Yes," Ken says. "A false join-up. Remember, now—Buddy's been chased in a round pen before. It can be scary for a horse; there's nowhere to go but around. And around." I hear Ken take a sip of coffee. "When he's coming to you in that video, it isn't out of free will; it's out of necessity, out of fear. Any port in a storm."

It is just like Ken to see the reality instead of my dream. Even the overused term *horse whisperer* repels him. For Ken, talking to horses is not some airy-fairy, new-age rite; it's honest, unsentimental exchange.

"Be careful next time. He might climb all over you," Ken tells me. And you can toss that clumsy big stick, too. All you need is a very light dressage whip, something more delicate and supple. It's just an extension of your arm anyway, not a bat."

I am crestfallen. Here I thought I'd found a slice of enlightenment, but even in a crude little video, Ken can see the truth.

"It's okay," Ken says before hanging up. "It's just that Buddy can't take the pressure yet. The round pen is already a place of discomfort for him. What you want ultimately is the horse to find you, not out of fear or desperation, but his own choice. Don't worry, your boy will be with you."

Chapter 7.

❦ *The Best Laid Plans* ❦

AT FIRST I DIDN'T TELL anyone about the baby. Not Sas, not my sister Rosemary, not even my mother. Coming from a family who tells one another just about everything, for me this was a radical departure, but I wanted Trey to be the first to know. And I wanted to tell him in person, but he was in Chicago fetching the last of his worldly possessions.

While I waited for his return, the familiar King James version of the nativity came to me, the one that Dad read every Christmas morning before we opened presents from under the tree. As kids, we thought that passage from the Gospel of Luke went on forever, but Mom—also a Mary—loved the part at the end when the mother of Jesus didn't go around making a big production about her pregnancy. She just "kept all these things and pondered them in her heart."

I, too, pondered these things in my heart. Who knew this could really happen? I was both elated and scared. Surely Mary must have had similar conflicted feelings, but then she was supposed to be carrying God. (Well, no wonder; I was carrying Zeus.)

I almost fainted when the little plastic device (oddly antiseptic for being the bearer of such earth-shattering information—the angel Gabriel it was not) confirmed what I'd instinctually known from the very first day: I'd conceived when Trey and I were in the Pacific Northwest.

It had been such a mythic road trip, starting with the Flory Ranch and then the drive to Washington. On the way up the coast I entertained Trey with more stories from my childhood home by the beach and all the animals we had there. The gardens and the pond with water lilies. "My only regret," I told him after we pulled out from a gas station, "is that you are not getting to see Meadowdale. How it was. I mean, that's the whole picture—the center of my family life." Mom and Dad had just moved to a condo in Kingston, a small harbor town across Puget Sound from our old Meadowdale house. Yes, the downsizing was easier for them, and all of us had our own lives now, but it was still hard for Paul, Rosemary, and me to say goodbye to the setting of our family history. I'd cried and cried when it sold. It felt like part of myself had disappeared.

"Yes, my sweet," Trey said. "But you're telling me about Meadowdale now. It's there in your heart. And in your memory and now in the stories you've been telling me since we met. Your horse. Your chickens. Dogs, cats, goats, your parakeet who chirped when he heard you trotting up the driveway on your horse!"

"I can't believe—you remember?" I said.

"Let's see..." Trey continued, clearing his throat..."Hens: Henny Penny? Clarabelle? Ah...Henrietta? Dogs: Captain and Muffin. Cats: hmmm...Sandy. Tinker? Mac, Franny, and Zooey. Can't remember all the others. Fish I can't remember at all, nor the bloody hamsters...But goats? Nanny and Lady. Oh! and Max the parakeet!"

Simply uttering the names of my beloved childhood animals brought Trey closer into the folds of my family, my intimate history.

"I know how you feel, though," he said, turning onto a northbound highway flocked by thick fir forests. "I so wish you could see my old family house, too. The estate in Dunbeath. My dad sold it after Mum died—on a whim—and moved to South America. The animals and everything—everything! It was all gone so quickly…At least you had time to say goodbye to your beloved home." Trey's mouth turned down. "Sometimes I wish I had Dunbeath myself. Of course, my sisters wanted it, too. But I would love for you to have seen it. Now it's owned by someone who has locked it up tight. There's no way we could go there. It's all changed anyway…"

"Well, then, you'd better tell *me* some more stories about Dunbeath," I said.

Trey then told me about the dog he'd raised as a puppy in his teens, a brown-and-white English setter.

"Trafalgar went everywhere with me, all over Dunbeath and beyond. He knew that land better than I did. Once I got lost with a hawk, and wandered from the moors into the wild wood, calling for her. It became late and I hadn't a clue where I was. Trafalgar stuck with me, and we finally found my falcon. Then he gently nosed me in the opposite direction and led me straight home."

I pictured Trey as boy with his precious dog so far from where I grew up. "Did Trafalgar like to play, too?" I asked, thinking of our dogs who were full of high hilarity.

"Yes," Trey said, slowing the car slightly. "Unlike some hunting dogs, Trafalgar was truly my friend. He went fishing with me, too, and never ever spooked the fish. He lived to see my own children." Trey paused, thoughts crowding his forehead. "Well, I've had a number of dogs since. But Trafalgar?" There was suddenly a catch in Trey's voice. "Trafalgar was different. He was faithful." I was moved by how Trey talked about his dog, but I found it strange that he seldom talked about his three teenage children who lived in Edinburgh with their mother on her family's estate. I made a mental note to ask Trey if we could invite them for Christmas.

"And when I was separated from my wife—before the divorce—I lived in a little rental—I think we could safely call it a hovel—Trafalgar was the only friend I really had." Trey's lips began to quiver. "And when he died," Trey caught his breath. "I thought I'd expire, too…" A lone tear made its way down Trey's cheek, then hung trembling under his chin.

It was a raucous homecoming. My brother, Paul, was home from Boston with his wife and new baby Catharine, and my sister, Rosemary, was eight months pregnant. I'd been so proud of Trey and the easy way he fit in. Much to my relief, he hadn't held forth too much. (My mother would often say to us as children, "Get in, say it, and get out!") All in all, Trey had passed the test, especially when he nabbed a salmon from Puget Sound for dinner. During the meal, my brother recited a poem by a Pacific Northwest poet about a river bird titled "The Water Ouzel," and Trey had answered, in full Scottish brogue, the famous Robert Burns poem:

> *…The best laid schemes of mice and men*
> *Go often askew,*
> *And leave us nothing but grief and pain,*
> *For promised joy!*

Everyone clapped. I took a big gulp of wine, relieved that Trey's recitation went over well, especially since my family was prone to heavy eye-rolling when confronted with poet-y bravado. If one of us strayed too close to the line, we were always quick to recall a scene when Paul and I were in our twenties, and he was a dorm master at Harvard, a job that helped pay for law school. One weekend when I was visiting, a particularly entitled freshman showed up at my brother's room shortly before midnight and flopped on the sofa, disheveled, as if laden with decades of artistic creation. With a huge sigh, dragging a stray hand through his mousse-mussed hair, he shook his head and said, "It's *hell* writing a novel."

If one of *us* got grandiose, there was even more eye-rolling, especially if it was me. When I was just out of college, all five of us were home for Christmas. Mom mentioned a new book she was devouring, *A Distant Mirror* by Barbara Tuchman. "Apparently the fourteenth century was a lot like our times," she said. "Economy, religious wars, a flourishing of art." My ears perked up. I was currently on a roll with mysticism. Meister Eckhart, Teresa of Avila, Julian of Norwich. I'd even considered applying to theological graduate school. I was searching for the ecstatic—even erotic—bliss of the seer. I wasn't quite sure if divinity school would provide me with such a vocation (where exactly *did* the mystics learn their trade?), but it was a start. I later abandoned the divinity school idea but was still entranced by Giotto, Chartres Cathedral, and troubadours. I had not read Mom's Barbara Tuchman, but I couldn't contain myself. In one sweeping statement (as if to claim Gregorian chant, the Book of Kells, and all of Britain's knights) I blurted, "Oh, I LOVE the Middle Ages!" Guffaws all around. I'd transgressed into the Kingdom of the Precious.

I was still on a high from the family visit when, on our drive back to Riojos, we approached a car that wasn't going as fast as Trey wanted it to. Since it was a treacherous, two-lane road along a winding river—and nighttime to boot—I trusted he'd be patient and wait till we'd emerged from the canyon. But he suddenly gunned right up behind the sedan and revved the motor. "Trey!" I said, and he laid his foot flat on the pedal, lurching us out into the oncoming traffic. "What are you doing!?" I said, grabbing the door handle as we nearly clipped the sedan's side mirror. To calm myself, I repeated the ancient Jesus Prayer over and over under my breath: "Lord Jesus Christ, son of God, have mercy upon me…Lord Jesus Christ have…" and we swerved back into our lane, barely avoiding an eighteen-wheeler.

"You have to look your fears in the face, Christine," Trey said, steadying the Trooper.

"What the fuck?" I could barely speak. That car's taillights were etched into my eyelids, the truck's bullhorn still bloating my ear-drums.

"Your fear will just get in the way if you don't confront it." His voice was edgy, weird, somebody else's voice. Then he dipped into a strange echoey chuckle, as if he'd just figured it out, "You can't hide from them. You just can't." I didn't know what to say. Part of me agreed with him. Our ongoing discussions about a life-truly-lived were always so energizing, how an artist has to go deeper every time. He'd often encouraged me to "punch through" to truth, whatever it was. Yes, I wanted to expand, to grow. Of course I needed to face my fears. (Didn't we all?) And no, I did not like to dwell on the ugly or nasty. (Who does?) But to purposely drive recklessly and say it was for my own good?

After a mile or so of deep and terrible silence, I finally said, "Trey…Why did this happen? Are you trying to prove something? If so, how can you risk *us?*" Even though the night was chilly on the mountain pass, I needed air. I cracked the window. My hands were still shaking.

After a few beats of silence, as if returning from a bad dream, Trey said, "I get wound up. I know. I know. And I know it isn't good for either of us…" His voice was his own again. "But to be honest, I just can't help myself. It's—it's like I'm being invaded by someone I can't get rid of." His face, flickering in the oncoming headlights, embodied the sweet Trey again. In a small voice he said, "Can you help me?"

"Of course," I said. "But first I'm taking over the driving. Pull over. Right now." I expected him to resist, but he quickly found a wide shoulder, pulled over, and stopped the car. We opened the doors, switched seats, and I pulled back onto the highway.

Taking the wheel calmed me. It gave me a better view of more than the highway. At first I didn't want to converse at all, but Trey was a man of words. And he used them so elegantly. Traveling in the dark is also a good way to say what we really feel, and soon Trey opened up more about his dad. "He taught me the vocabulary of cruelty," he said. "Sometimes it just comes out."

After another stretch of silence, he said, "I don't want to botch it up this time; I want to keep you. No catch-and-release for us. You are the only true thing in my life." Though flattering, this "one true thing" was a lot to carry. I wondered if his former girlfriend in Chicago (apparently, she left without taking anything, including her car) was as crazy as he made her out to be.

But each time we wrestled with his demons, we reached what he called a "new weir." It felt like growing, like progress, even if it took some time to recover. As we wended our way south, I also reminded myself that Trey had had a pretty crummy deal as a kid. An absent mother who died when he was a teenager, a talented narcissistic father, and an isolated childhood with tutors and the occasional nanny. I'd read that few women can resist falling for a motherless boy.

"I have to admit," Trey said as I downshifted for a curve, "meeting your family made me kind of envious. Your brother, your sister—you all have an unspoken bond with your parents. You actually laugh with them. They know your stories. You know theirs. They listen to you. I don't think I've ever felt that. Ever…"

"Well, what did your dad do exactly?" I asked cautiously.

"You don't want to know the half of it," Trey said.

"Well, maybe if you tell me a little more it will help," I said, glad for a place to direct the problem. Tiny house lights far in a field twinkled in the distance as the Trooper sliced its way through the dark.

"Let's put it this way," Trey said. "Dad was not exactly patient. I told you about his disgust with my riding ability. But even when we were little—well, once when my sister was a baby—in actual fact, it's the only time I can recall my dad holding her—she reached for his martini. I suppose the shiny glass attracted her, but she wanted the red chili pepper. Dad pulled it right out of his drink and fed it to her. I will never forget her screams. Or my dad laughing."

Trey said there were so many times he was disappointed his father he couldn't count them, but one was still vivid. When he was six, he'd been afraid of the dark, and one night he'd called out for his mom. Receiving no answer, he stumbled into his parents' bedroom to find his father, midcoitus, with a woman Trey didn't know. "Get Out! Get the hell out now!" his father had screamed. "Don't you know any better?!"

By the time we got back to Riojos, we had indeed made it to new weir, closer (and wiser), I thought. Trey's chilling stories about his father that night stuck with me, though. Such behavior was miles apart from my experience with my own father.

When I was six, I'd gone through a protracted phase of believing witches lived in my bedroom closet. Convinced they were in the basement, too, I sneaked to the freezer when Mom asked me to fetch the ice cream. But upstairs, in my bed tucked under the eaves, I thought for sure I heard the ones in my closet scratching behind my headboard. So my father, in his practical way, rigged up a spring-latched lock on my closet door. Each night before we said prayers, together we turned on the closet lights to check for witches, then secured the door tightly. "See? You just lock this," he'd said, demonstrating how the spring latch prevented the hook from opening. "Those witches cannot come out."

With Trey, as with other close friends who'd endured violent or traumatic childhoods, I harbored a certain responsibility to help because my parents gave me not only love, but confidence that the world was mine to delight in. Couldn't my family show Trey the way?

Of course, friends and boyfriends would sometimes poke fun at my family, even though they, too, were drawn in. "Norman Rockwell!" my Boston boyfriend said once, which made me cringe. Granted, cheer was a known commodity in the Hemp Family (it helped keep the demons at bay), but the truth was, we actually *liked* being together.

When I was eight, I climbed the huge birch tree in Meadowdale— to the top, a big victory (I could see all the way to Whidbey Island). I'd raced in to tell Mom. "Oh, I'd love to do that with you!" she said, hugging me tight. Though she never did climb that tree, her enthusiasm for my adventures didn't wane. Right after college, when I took a job in Vermont as a rough carpenter, Mom asked over the phone, "How are you doing at that hammer place?" I rolled my eyes, "Mom—it's more than a 'hammer place'!" I told her about shimmying up to the barn rafters to shingle the roof, the foreman's call for "coffee time!" and how I'd bought yet another tool for my toolbox: "A bevel square!" I told her proudly.

Picking up the phone and calling my mother was always a given, a luxury I couldn't imagine living without. At 24, when I'd landed my first job as a schoolteacher in rural New Hampshire, I called her after the first day of teaching seven—yes, seven—sections of sophomore English, earning me a whopping $8,500 a year with a $100 bonus to direct all the school plays.

"Well? Tell me everything," she said. In my family, when we're emotionally, intellectually, or socially drained—even for good reasons—we say, "I have to take a shower now!" I told her yes, I definitely had to take a shower now.

I phoned Mom often to keep her up to speed with the details of my little school and how, in Vermont/New Hampshire, they say cool things like "I'm goin' downt' Haverill"—no matter *where* Haverhill is. Everything is always "downt'." I told her about buying fresh milk in a tin jug at a nearby farm, and how my students awoke at 3:00 a.m. to milk those cows. I also told her about the day Steve Robby had mouthed off and rabble-roused one time too many. I'd reached the tipping point and finally demanded that my whole class of sophomores put their heads on their desks, close their eyes, be quiet, and "just think about things" (clearly a last resort). I sat for the rest of the class period at my desk (tears in my eyes) pretending to grade papers but writing a poem instead. When the bell rang, Teresa Clark, the quietest girl in the school, slipped by my desk on her way out and dropped a handwritten note, one I've saved to this day: "Miss Hemp: You are muchmuchmuchmuchmuchmuch more than anyone can imagine." I decided to keep on teaching.

Finally, Mom couldn't stay away any longer, so on my spring break week she flew east to see things for herself. One Saturday in March, we explored the Connecticut River Valley, looking for the house of Donald Hall, an author we admired, especially his poem titled "Names of Horses," which touched both of us in its fierce and loving litany of his grandfather's teams, long dead, who had shouldered everything from plowing to taking the family to church on Sundays:

> ...*old toilers, soil makers:*
> *Oh, Roger, Mackerel, Riley, Ned, Nellie, Chester, Lady*
> *Ghost...*

He'd also written a memoir titled *String Too Short to Be Saved*, an account of moving back to live in his grandparents' house where he'd spent his boyhood summers. On the front cover of the book, a daguerreotype of his eighteenth-century house charmed those of us who'd grown up on the shores of Puget Sound, where "old" houses seldom predate the 1920s. An hour or so of winding through New England hamlets brought us to the village of Andover. At the post office we spilled out of the car and asked the postmaster which way to Wilmot. He laughed, "What are you looking for?" Sheepishly we told him that we wanted to see Donald Hall's house, the one on the cover of his book.

"Oh! Don would love to see you! Why don't I give him a call?"

"No!" we protested. "We only want to see the house." The prospect of a human encounter was more than we could contemplate, but the postmaster already had the poet on the line.

"Don! There are a couple of ladies here who would love to stop by and see you. Uh-huh. Sure!" He hung up and grinned. "He says come over right away. He's expecting you for tea." My mother and I gasped but didn't want to appear ungrateful. We thanked the postmaster and climbed back into the car nervous and giggly, then followed his directions to Hall's house.

Hall waved as we pulled to a stop. "Hello!" he said. "Call me Don." We told him our names, taking in his large, furry beard, and smiling face. "Welcome!" he said, helping Mom with the car door. Hall's wife, Jane Kenyon, waved from the garden. Hall introduced us, then ushered us into the living room where wide, smooth floorboards creaked under our footsteps.

Hall learned that I was an aspiring poet. "What are you working on now?" he asked, and I thought of the tattered drafts scattered across my makeshift desk, a door on two sawhorses. "Oh...," I said, blanking out. Same as when I'm asked to name my favorite novel, the only book I can ever remember reading is *Stormy, Misty's Foal*.

"I'm working on poems, yes...but I'm not sure that they're worth anything," I confessed. He suddenly leaped up out of his chair and bounded up the narrow stairs. Mom and I exchanged glances as we heard him rummaging around in the room above us. Soon he came down with a shiny new book about the craft of writing. "Here. I'll sign it for you!" he said. I thanked him profusely. This was all so exciting I could hardly wait for it to be over so I could go home and think about it.

"I've just been to see my good friend James Wright," Hall said as he settled back in his chair and took a slurp of tea. "He has throat cancer and can no longer talk or eat through his mouth." Mom and I leaned forward, remembering it was James Wright who wrote the poem Mom had clipped from a magazine and tucked into my bedroom mirror the first Thanksgiving I came home from college. "A Blessing" recounts stopping on a highway and encountering two horses in a field at dusk. Their soft muzzles welcome him, and they "bow shyly as wet swans." I'd always been especially moved by the last lines, and it occurred to me there in Donald Hall's living room that they mirrored my feelings at that very moment:

> *...Suddenly I realize*
> *That if I stepped out of my body I would break*
> *Into blossom.*

Hall told us about his friendship with Wright and how, even without being able to speak, Wright's poetic voice was still intact. "He's sitting in his hospital bed," Hall explained. "And he looks terrible. I sit next to him on the bed and I think how awful this is. What can I say? But he manages to write me a note. 'Don,' it says, 'I'm dying,' and then he stops and looks up at me." Hall's eyes are bright. "I am speechless. What can I say? Then. In his inimitable genius for line breaks, Jim writes me another line: 'to eat ice cream from a tray.'" Hall let out a deep breath, leaned back into his chair, and grinned. "Isn't that great?"

When we finished our tea and cookies it was time to go, and Mom and I, fearful of overstaying our welcome, thanked him and waved goodbye. Once we were safely in the car and pointed west to Vermont, my mother said, "I have to take a shower now." I agreed. "He was even nice to the *mother*," Mom said, rolling down the window to let in the cold, spring air. I gave my car some gas to tackle the uphill grade.

"Poet-finding," Mom said, remembering the "stud-finding" excursions during my horse days. The 4-H girls would spend a Saturday checking out stallions for possible breeding of their mares. Though my horse Lightfoot was an Arabian gelding, Mom and I often went on these local trips. We'd nearly collapsed when the club leader, Mrs. Clark, would say, in all seriousness, "Today is a good stud-finding day."

"Today, the poet-finding was good," Mom said, and we headed toward my home, crossing the Swiftwater covered bridge, which spans the Wild Ammonoosuc River. The wooden crosspieces clunk-clunked as I slowed down, and the surface of the river, still covered with ice, was crisscrossed with dark cracks. We pulled over and walked down along the bank.

"Listen," Mom said. And like some primordial groan, the river began to talk. First deep creaking, then cracks like thunder and lightning made us jump and step back. Blue chunks buckled and broke in front of us, slowly churning and inching downstream. Like fingernails scratching a blackboard, the sound was both crazy-making and thrilling, as if memory and prescience were colliding. Then the ice cracked all the way across to the other bank. Rocks emerged from underneath and the chunks piled against them in a dam while other bergs smashed past. We watched the water take the ice far downstream over riffles and around the bend, on its way to melting them into nothing. If we stepped out of our bodies, I thought, we might just blossom.

When Trey returned from Chicago and found out that his gods had had their way, he was ecstatic. I'd kept it secret from the family for almost a month, but finally I couldn't wait any longer.

"Mom, I'm going to have a baby," I said to her over the phone. I stood in the kitchen, the window framing an early snowfall, flakes coming down in puffs on the pink adobe buildings.

"Oh, Christine, your baby will be so loved," she said.

"Do you think it will be all right, Mom?"

"The baby?"

"Yes, the baby."

"Of course," she said, evaporating all my doubts. "Why wouldn't it? You are healthy and strong. Hey, what if you gave yourself a little break from work if you can. Can you take on fewer projects right now? You have a tendency to cram a lot of stuff in. Why not leave some time blank on your calendar if you can. Trey will help, won't he?"

I knew Trey was hopeless with domestic things like cooking, and he told me once that he and his wife had had "help" with their children. He was so excited about this child, though, and told me again and again we would do this together.

"Take a bath." Mom said. "Read a little more. Sit with Badger and Callie. Make some popcorn in the evenings." We both laughed, knowing how popcorn was such a bright spot for both of us. "This is the time you can be truly selfish," she said.

I was banking on Trey's help, even though he didn't seem to know much about infants. But Mom's reassurance helped to push away any fears that lingered about having a child so late. Mom had had us in her late twenties and early thirties, and I'd just turned 40. This was clearly my last shot at having a family.

"You won't be alone with this, you know," she said. "I will come down, and Rosemary will, too. We'll just cozy up together with that baby!" I hung up the phone, picturing the three of us—or four since Rosemary was due any day—nestled on the couch with Zeus.

The day after that conversation, Rosemary called at the crack of dawn to report that she'd just given birth to Celia Rose.

"She weighs six pounds, thirteen ounces," Rosemary said. "And I feel much lighter."

I repeated the unusual name: "Celia! Celia Rose!? What color hair does she have?"

"Blonde! Just like you!" Rosemary said. "And a lot of it!"

"Well, I've got some news, as well…," I said.

Soon my whole family was excited about my baby. Paul called from Boston. "Hey! Catharine is certainly getting cousins quickly! She'll be glad about that." Whatever reservations Mom may have had about Trey or my pregnancy, she cheered me on, as always. "You will be a terrific mother," she said. "Just think of how good you were with Lightfoot."

Chapter 8.

～Blood Sports ～

AS CHRISTMAS APPROACHED, MY BELLY grew. "You're joining the 'Hut'!" Rosemary said over the phone, referring to a term coined by her friend Kelly, a mother of three who praised the connection among women preparing for childbirth. Sas, a mother of two grown girls, made me a many-layered painting of Madonnas. "You are going to be the mother of men!" she said, holding up her colorful piece with a flourish. I felt like I was being accepted into a private club, one that seemed to exclude men, or at least relegate them to a sidebar. Usually this would have offended me—the tomboy, carpenter, fly-fisherman, friend-of-many-men. Instead I felt fecund and sensual. Tribal.

"I wonder what the poor people are doing today?" Trey asked me one November morning with a sweet smile, referring to the riches of our love. He held me carefully, and I wondered if our baby would have his dark hair and upturned mouth.

A couple weeks later, I was teaching a three-day workshop for scientists at Los Alamos. The National Laboratory hired me regularly to help physicists as well as administrators with their writing and communication skills; it provided a good chunk of change, something Trey and I would need with the baby on its way. At the end of day two, I returned to my B & B and discovered spotting, little flecks of blood. I lay on the bed not knowing what to do. I put my feet up and tried to dismiss it as a normal part of pregnancy, but my heart raced, and by nighttime the flow was more than a few spots.

"I'm bleeding," I told Trey shakily over the phone.

"Oh, I've seen this before, darling," he said. "It's nothing to worry about. It happened with two of my kids. It'll stop. Trust me. Just breathe." I took a breath and held it.

"I just hope Zeus is okay in there," I said, trying to keep our shared delight alive.

"He'll be fine. Our baby wouldn't desert us," he said. "Just hang in there. You are so strong and so is Zeus." I hung up less agitated, but I didn't dare get to my feet. I stayed in bed, hoping that the bleeding would subside. I read (yet again) the chapter about spotting in *What to Expect When You're Expecting*, a book Rosemary had sent, and I'd kept it right by my side ever since. In the morning the flow was heavier. I taught my entire class sitting down with my legs crossed, a pad collecting blood.

After the long drive home on dark, icy roads, I already knew what the doctor would later tell me. I wept without reserve and lay in bed sobbing so loudly that Badger and Callie jumped up and cried, too. The next morning, Trey brought me a latte in bed, "Well, the good news is you can drink wine and caffeine now."

This seemed a small consolation, but it was sweet of him to say nonetheless. "It's just so sad," I wept again. "Zeus was there and now he isn't? I just don't know what to do." Trey leaned toward me and brushed my hair aside.

"You'll get pregnant again. No question. We are fertile people," he said and wrapped me in his arms. I spent the next few days in a stupor.

But I couldn't stay in such a state because two of Trey's children were due in ten days for Christmas. Lena, fifteen, and Morland, seventeen. His youngest son, James, had decided to stay home with his mother. I had food to prepare and cleaning to do. Thinking the baby would be well along, we had planned our first real "family Christmas."

Trey was twitchy anticipating his children's arrival, as if losing Zeus meant that I might leave him, too. But I'd planned on taking Trey's children to the little adobe Episcopal church for Christmas Eve service. I'd bought advent calendars and presents for both teenagers. Trey and I decided not to tell his children about Zeus. In the days that followed, I dragged out cookbooks and pored over advice on how to cook turkey. I figured out how long a twenty-two-pound bird would have to sit in my tiny oven. Sas came over with instructions for gravy, and I learned a new word, *roux*, which I pictured as being spelled "rue," fitting with my mood. When I suddenly broke into tears and hunched over the kitchen counter, Sas rubbed my back softly. I continued to sob while clutching her gravy recipe.

That afternoon I decorated the house with evergreens, noting the aching in my arms, something new since the miscarriage. My therapist, Lewis, had told me that this was not uncommon after the loss of a child, that one's limbs are missing what they once held, or were meant to hold. So, while Trey was picking up his kids at the airport in Albuquerque, I went out and carried in a stack of piñon wood and lit a fire in the huge kiva fireplace, hoping the kids would like the unique aroma of a Taos fire. And I hung stockings. Soon I heard the Trooper pull in just as it was beginning to snow. I watched from the window as they tumbled out of the car. Lena clearly had Trey's nose and cheekbones. Morland had his tall stature. "Wow!" Morland said as he politely stomped the snow off his shoes and held out his hand. "This is beautiful. Hello, Christine. Thank you for inviting us." Well-bred accent.

"And I'm Lena," the girl said, her hair shyly swinging in front of her smiling face. I hugged them both and brought them all in by the fire. When Sas and her partner, John, just in from Berkeley, invited us over for a cookie-decorating party, we gladly accepted. Sas was trying to make things easier for me, so we all tromped through the snow next door to her casita. After pulling many sheets of cookies out of the oven, we began with colored sprinkles and chocolate frosting. John casually asked us what we were having for Christmas dinner.

Trey laughed a strange laugh he channeled from some distant, empty compartment, "Well, if Christine doesn't burn the damned thing, we're having turkey!" The guttural quality of the chuckle contorted his mouth. Both Lena and Morland flinched in the middle of decorating a gingerbread boy, as if their bodies could tell the story out loud. The room instantly got quiet. No one said a thing. Both John and Sas knew what I'd been through the previous week and couldn't meet my eyes. My humiliation was more intense as the moment expanded into the air around us, cookies left undecorated and no one knowing what to say. I felt as if a hot poker had been rammed into my belly. Soon the party broke up and the kids took a walk in the field behind the Rocking H.

"This cannot happen again," I told Trey that night when we were alone.

"I can't help myself," he pleaded. "It just comes out." He apologized as I sank into bed and scooted far over to the edge. But he was right. He couldn't help himself. The next evening after dinner Lena and I were making a pumpkin pie and Trey was putting up the tree we'd bought that afternoon. Morland was reading, his legs swung gracefully over the couch arm. "This is the best Christmas we've ever had, Dad," he looked up from his book. "It's happy here."

"Where's the wrench?" Trey snapped, and we all jumped. Morland put down his book. Trey held up the metal stand, its one leg dangling off the base like that of an injured cat. I scrambled to find the toolbox, and Lena stepped back into the kitchen.

"Where did you get this stand?" He awkwardly tried to push the screw out of the tray. Then he threw down the hammer. I backed up toward Lena, her face glazed over. Morland got up and headed toward his dad's casita.

I took the pie out of the oven. "Come on, Lena," I said. "Let's go to the hardware store to get a new one." We rode together in silence, fully aware of our complicity in Trey's behavior. I felt like a spectator in my own drama and I didn't know how to stop the play. And my arms ached. Lena and I found another stand, one that did not require assembling, and on the way home she told me she loved the halibut I'd made for dinner. I reached over and held her hand. She squeezed mine back, and for a moment we could have been mother and daughter.

After the children left, Trey was less twitchy, but when he was, I had the distinct impression that what I was building with him would crumble if I didn't dash around to catch the mortar and cram it back between the bricks. It almost seemed as if losing Zeus made him afraid he'd lose everything. One friend assured me that Trey was grieving in his own way, and this was bound to happen with any couple. My friends talked all the time about their partners or husbands who had been selfish or thoughtless. Sometimes I thought maybe I was just a wimp, spoiled by a family who did not cotton to conflict.

I finally asked Paul. Since childhood my brother has had my back. When I was six and Paul was ten, his pal Doug Mogal had purposely scribbled—with my brand-new colored felt pens—all through my special sketchbook. I was devastated. In tears I showed it to Paul, and he promptly sent Doug packing and was never asked back. In junior high, he drove (with a fresh driver's license) across town to rescue me from a party that was much wilder than I had prepared for, keeping my phone call to him a secret from our parents. He talked me through high school and college boyfriend troubles. My brother's allegiance is like the law of gravity. He knew I'd never given or risked as much as I had with Trey. So after telling him about Trey's short temper after the miscarriage, Paul asked outright, "Well, is it worth it? Does the good outweigh the bad with Trey? If you had to list all the good and all the bad, which comes out ahead?"

Paul's questions made my relationship with Trey seem like a math problem. I appreciated that my brother didn't tell me what to do or pass judgment. He might have wondered if Trey was really the man for me, but the thing is, I did not wonder. I was already in. I had made that commitment in my mind and heart, and I believed in riding it out, no matter what. Plus, I didn't see myself as a person who would choose a less than honorable man. In a way I suppose I considered myself already married. I had carried his child. This was it. Didn't my long-term coupled friends—both straight and gay— tell me how hard it was sometimes? Working out big emotional differences, and even daily things like doing the dishes? This was the first time I'd thrown in the big saddlebag. Having made that decision, my heart was set. The rest was the dance of merging and adjusting and creating. This was the part I was prepared to roll up my sleeves for.

After all, Trey and I were so well matched. The delight we took in each other's work, the way we looked at the world, even break-fast conversation was fortified with inquiry, hilarity, and surprise. A mere cup of coffee could evolve into rumination about the history of domesticity or a meditation on poetry. "Or doggerel!" Trey might say, which always cracked us up.

Right after I hung up with my brother, Trey came home with groceries, put his arm around me and held me tight. "Why not let's drive to Santa Fe this afternoon and have dinner? Beforehand, we can pop into that parrot shop?" I loved that place, especially the parrot named Scud, who squawked "Let me outta here!" I ran to get my coat.

I realized then that my brother's pro-and-con scale weighed in way more strongly on the pro side. And after Christmas Trey had even agreed to see my therapist, Lewis, both with me and alone. In the months that followed there were huge changes. He started listening if I called him on his moods, and he even suggested we practice Pema Chodron's meditation about lovingkindness.

Fortified by Lewis and practices to fall back on, Trey settled into the Rocking H as if it were his long-lost homestead. In his endearingly clumsy way, he built a frame for compost in the garden; we worked, we fly-fished, and we made new friends, threw dinner parties (champagne in the tub), and planned for our future. Juan, too, thoroughly enjoyed Trey's enthusiasms—not only fly-fishing, but talking novels and politics. Juan told me Trey and I were "a wholesome couple."

So when an invitation came for me to teach a workshop in London, it made sense that Trey would come, too. He'd do some book dealing in the city and then he wanted to show me his old haunts in Scotland. There also was talk of fly-fishing for Atlantic salmon, but the main destination was a hunting lodge in the Highlands where all his falconer friends gathered every fall.

Though he'd written off falconry, he was eager to introduce me to his hawking friends. I was more than willing; the sport seemed so elegant and full of pageantry like the falconry books he collected and sold. Many of his antique books were embossed in gold leaf, and the colored illustration plates of falcons, gauntlets, and hoods evoked the world of medieval knights. The art dates back 3,000 years to the Mongols, who hunted game birds along the Steppes. And Arabs, too, practiced it long before it came to Europe, riding their horses across the dunes, releasing their hawks mid-gallop.

In the many months since the miscarriage, I hadn't been able to get pregnant again, so the trip to Britain seemed like a perfect antidote. I also was eager to tell my mother about my upcoming adventure, remembering the spring she and I had explored England together. Mom had flown from Seattle to London, and we set off from where I lived and taught school near Windsor. That particular journey with Mom remained one of our favorites, despite the fact that my flat had no heat. It was so chilly we could see our breath indoors. I'd had to pry her out of the down comforter in her bed.

"The car will be warm, Mom. Promise," I told her. I was glad I'd rented a car, that we weren't risking the expedition in my (drafty) Volkswagen bug, which had to be started on an incline. We planned to drive north to Shropshire and Derbyshire to track A. E. Houseman and the Brontë sisters. Mom wanted to poke around Jane Austen's Bath, too, and we had reservations at a B & B in a little village called Diddlebury ("an unfortunate name!" as my father would say).

The morning after her arrival, Mom ventured into my frigid kitchen. "This lettuce is frozen," she said, picking it up from the counter. Though my living room had a view out to the footpath to Prune Hill (which led to the Magna Carta signing site) and horses grazed in the field beyond, it wasn't exactly cozy. My hot water heater was roughly the size of a cooking pot. To take a bath I had to supplement the bathwater by heating the electric kettle and pouring in six or eight potfuls to make even a tepid bath. When I climbed into the huge cast-iron tub, I'd lie down flat on my back, arms to my sides, and splash three inches of water on my body like a seal flapping in a tide pool.

I was eager to get Mom on the road so she wouldn't have to endure the tub.

"You can't live this way," Mom said, after a trip downstairs to the Thorpe Store for fresh bread and fruit for the trip. "Period. Paragraph."

We motored off toward Hertfordshire to visit friends of friends, an English architect and his wife expecting us for dinner. We anticipated the encounter with mild apprehension, not unlike our introduction to Donald Hall. We didn't know these people either, but my friends insisted we go see them. Apparently, they were delightful, and at least it would be an interesting house, remodeled from a Norman structure. When we had finally found it, we were glad to end the day's journey. Our hostess opened the door with a radiant smile. "Please do come in!" she said as we made our way toward the living room festooned with Laura Ashley fabric and contemporary furniture.

"But I must tell you straightaway," she said. "Something terrible has happened." We paused. "Our heat has gone on the blink, I'm afraid."

Mom and I exchanged brief glances.

"Oh! That's okay!" we protested, our eyes casing the joint for anything that resembled a blanket or stove. Our hostess showed us to our room, where sumptuous down comforters and hot water bottles were at the ready, a relief to us both. When we came out for drinks, our host had lit a fire in the large, stone fireplace. He was flapping a newspaper at the gasping little flames. Not exactly a roaring blaze, but we moved closer, shivering as the monks must have done at the nearby fourteenth-century abbey. I knew Mom was counting the minutes till we could retreat to those down comforters. Finally, after a delicious soup with our hosts, and thanking them from our hearts, we headed straight to our beds.

Right before sinking into sleep, my mother's voice rose in the dark, "I just love the Middle Ages."

The writing workshop in London happened to fall on the weekend following Princess Diana's funeral, an event that aroused a collective, public grief I'd never before experienced. People on the streets sobbed openly, and on the day of the funeral the entire city was silent, everyone glued to their televisions. Her sudden death was blamed on the paparazzi who, like predators, tailed her car at high speed through a Paris tunnel. Diana's driver, intent on ditching them, lost control of the vehicle, and the rest is history.

After a week in the city, Trey was more than eager to leave London and all its grieving. As our plane lifted off from Heathrow to Inverness, out the window we could see mountains of bouquets piled outside Kensington Palace. "I really don't know what all the kerfuffle is about. I met Diana once," he said, pulling the flight magazine from the seat pocket. "She was just another Sloane Ranger." I chalked up Trey's crude remark to the stress of traveling and settled into my seat. Once we landed in Inverness and headed out in our rental car, things brightened. "Isn't this splendid?" he said as we made our way through the undulating moors, their greens, grays and buff-colored hills fading into the crevices of the Highlands. He pointed to a marvelous stag looking our way. "I used to stalk here," he said, and told me about his hunting trips every fall. "It's why my right ear is deaf." He laughed. "I've had enough of shooting."

With London obligations behind us, we were now free to have our own adventure. Scotland opened up, and September sun warmed the hills. As we pulled into a B & B for the night, I asked him where we were going fishing.

"Ah!" he smiled and reached over to touch my cheek. "You just wait, darling. We're going to the River Forss." The next day I found out he had secretly hired a ghillie for a beautiful beat, a private section of river on which he was authorized to guide. Trey speycast his line at an angle to the current and I just used my heavier Sage trout rod, but each of us landed an Atlantic salmon, something the ghillie said was a first that year. "She's the real fisherman!" Trey told him, grinning and proud. We fished the pools and curves of this tea-colored Scottish river through the afternoon, stashed our salmon in a cooler with ice, then headed deeper into the Highlands.

"Before we meet the falconers," Trey said, reaching across to touch my shoulder, "I want to introduce you to someone."

"Who could that be?" I asked.

"I wanted to surprise you. I have told her all about you. She and her husband used to let me fly my hawks on her land. You'll love her. Her name is Enrica. She's actually...well, Mrs. Macbeth!" He laughed freely and sweetly. "And I've so wanted her to meet you! I couldn't wait to surprise you." He rocked back and forth at the steering wheel, his body at home in this rugged country, his face beaming. "But we have to change clothes before we get there. We're invited for dinner and to spend the night."

"We're spending the night in her house?"

He turned off onto a narrow road lined by hedgerows. "It's more a castle, actually."

"What does one wear to dinner at Macbeth's castle?" I asked, glad I'd packed a skirt at the last minute.

"Nothing that will show red spots, I should think," Trey said with a poker face and a twinkle in his eye. Apparently, the Thane of Cawdor had died several years earlier, but the Countess still lived in the fourteenth-century Cawdor Castle snuggled next to the forest at Nairn, the very setting of Shakespeare's play. We stopped along the way on a wooded road, and I slipped into black tights, a short, gray skirt, and a sky-blue turtleneck. Trey put on a clean shirt. He always seemed to buy shirts and jackets that were too small for his frame. He hadn't a clue how large a man he really was, his arms sticking out below his cuffs. We arrived a bit early, so Trey suggested we walk through the grounds of Cawdor Castle. I took his arm and we meandered through the forest. As we got farther along the path, it was easy to picture three witches in the clearing, busy with their toiling and troubling. I was glad to get back out into the sunshine.

When we strolled in the Castle's summer residence, we were met by a slim, glamorous woman of about sixty with auburn hair, piercing green eyes, and an elegant gait. "Lady Cawdor!" Trey said, opening his arms with warmth and fondness.

"Welcome!" she said and hugged Trey back. "This must be your beloved! How wonderful you two look together! Trey, why don't you have Martin show you where to put your bags. Oh, do come see my gardens," she said, taking me by the hand. She and I strolled through the knot garden with its elegant geometric shapes. Aromatic plants and herbs were pruned into delicate sculptures, and we sat in the grass and faced the banks of late summer gladiolas and cosmos in the warm September sun. She said she always had loved wild animals, perhaps because of her childhood in Rhodesia. But once when her Scottish husband, the Thane, was still alive, there had been a hunting party at the Castle. They'd shot a lot of migrating geese for sport, and the gunshots had tortured her, just hearing the geese falling and falling.

"That night," she said, "a lone goose kept flying back here." She pointed up. "In circles. Searching and searching for its lost mate. They mate for life, you know." The Countess tipped her head, as if listening again for that sad sound. "It called and called…" Tears welled up in her eyes and I felt a lump in my own throat, my baby-loss so fresh and raw.

"I finally told my husband, 'Sweetheart, go out there now and shoot that poor bird. It's too sad. I cannot bear its loneliness and grief any longer.'" She began to weep, the autumn sun slanting across her castle keep. Drawn into her sudden grief, I watched the Countess in the waning light, childless and without her mate, and wondered if her loneliness was like Princess Diana's. Women isolated in a social class that didn't allow much outward expression. As if she'd read my thoughts, the Countess suddenly got up briskly and said, "Shall we get ready for supper then? I'll let you pick and arrange the flower bouquet for the table."

Trey appeared and said he'd given our fresh salmon to Martin, the chef, who was baking it with herbs from the garden. The aroma wafted in as we gathered in a small dining room festooned with candles. Martin floated by with hot plates and served the fish at the table with vegetables from the garden. He called the Countess "M'Lady," pouring each of us a crisp Sauterne and then left the room. The evening stretched on with a delicious chocolate mousse and cognac while portraits of the family forebears stared down at us. Middle Ages all over the place. I couldn't wait to tell my mother.

The next day Trey was making calls and plans to meet the falconers, so the Countess invited me to spend the day with her. We zoomed off across the moors in her Land Rover, stopping so she could show me a secret glade where every year she picked chanterelles. We collected a basketful, then toured the vast expanse of land that belonged to the castle. The undulating moors seemed to go on and on. Every so often the Countess would stop at a gate, get out of the car, and sort through the countless keys jangling on a huge ring she snapped to her belt. I wondered what she was locking out or locking in. Then she'd unbolt another gate so we could drive another ten kilometers.

"See there?" she slowed and pointed to a herd of deer looking our way. "No more hunting on my land. My husband used to let Trey fly his hawks here," she turned to me and downshifted. "But as you can tell, I'm not keen on the blood sports. I want this to be a safe haven for animals now." She slowed for a grouse awkwardly flapping its way across the dirt track.

"Trey is taking me to meet the falconers," I said cautiously. "He wants me to see what used to consume so much of his time. At least he tells it this way—I guess it was a kind of manic passion?" The Countess maneuvered around a huge pothole in the road, her back straight and lips pursed, as if the subject left no room for comment.

We drove back to the castle in silence, passing the trail where Trey and I had lost our way.

When Trey and I left Cawdor late that afternoon, our bags full of tartan scarves and seeds from the Cawdor garden, the Countess said to Trey, "Now don't you dare let her get away; she's better than any hawk!"

"Oh, I know, Enrica," Trey said, kissing the Countess on both cheeks. "I have no intention of losing her," and he pulled me close.

At the lodge we were greeted by a dozen falconers and their wives and girlfriends. Lots of shouting and slapping of backs. "Trey!! Great to see you, lad! Is this your fiancée you've been telling us about?" "Yes!" he said, draping his arm around my shoulder and introducing me to everyone. Trey was relaxed and himself, his eyes bright. A fire blazed in the mammoth fireplace, and old tapestries hung in the spacious living room. Pointers and spaniels lay about the floor in front of the fire. The falconers ranged from a shack-dwelling bachelor to an Italian count. After dinner we drank whiskey by the fire, and I rested my hand on Trey's thigh as he entertained them all with stories of the Rocking H, our life in New Mexico, and how he'd finally found his true home. He turned to me, his face radiant. "This," he said, grinning at me, "is the love of my life! She is my true north!" Everyone said "Ohhh!" and "How wonderful for you both!" and the dogs jerked awake briefly then flopped their heads back down on their paws.

The next morning after a big breakfast, we all trudged across the moor. Deer scat lay in the grass, and tiny birds huddled on a branch of a lone fir. Some of the men (but mostly the wives) carried cadges, over-the-shoulder racks for the hooded falcons. The birds bobbed and swayed, their talons gripping the perches, their decorative leather hoods like quail plumes.

"Quite a few of these falconers have lost their wives," Trey said.

"They died?" I asked, pulled up short from admiring Trey in his Wellington boots, tweed jacket, and buoyant spirits.

"Oh, no," he laughed. "The women just left. See James there?" He pointed to a man carrying his own birds. "His girlfriend told him enough was enough. Everything revolved around the hawks. He told me she left him a couple of months ago." A slight breeze rustled the birch trees, their yellow leaves still hanging on. A shadow flitted across his face, as if he were holding something back from me. Maybe about his ex-wife. I wondered if he could be counted among those falconers who lost their mates.

"See? See?" Trey giggled and whispered, cultivating collusion with me as we followed the wives and the falconers. "I used to do this," he admitted. "All the time. To the point of not coming home even. Once I lost my favorite falcon and I was out all night searching." Trey got quiet. "I finally found her, but she was starving. When I fed her, she gorged so much that she was too weak to digest it. Her death never should have happened." Another cloud brushed across his face.

The dogs began to whine. The falconers kept them on a tight leash, which seemed to make them even more restless, their tongues lolling out and their noses reaching toward an invisible scent. The falcons, on the other hand, reminded me of soldiers patiently waiting for battle. They rocked and traveled calmly on the cadges. Trey explained the wind, the landscape, and how "Everything has to be just right. Or it can go terribly wrong." The words "terribly wrong" would not leave my ears. I tried to imagine what that would be. Trey was intent on showing me this sport, but he made fun of it as well—which made me feel safer, but it also betrayed some fierce tug-of-war between his two worlds.

The party stopped near a rise where an old crag from a fallen tree lay on the ground. The wind touched our faces, and a feeling of anticipation ran through the group, including the dogs who strained even more on their leashes, their whines frantic. The Italian count, ready for his first flight of the day, unleashed his quivering pointer. In a flash the brown dog was gone, straight toward a nearby copse where he circled and shook, trying to track the scent of grouse. Meanwhile, the Count removed the hood from his falcon's head. Its talons clutched his leather gauntlet. The bird's head pivoted almost all the way around, eyes cold and yellow. Considering the moor, the sky, the ruckus around the grove of bushy trees without any visible emotion, she began to stretch her mottled, powerful wings.

"Now," Trey whispered to me and his fingers shook. "He's giving her the go-ahead." The Count raised his arm higher, and the falcon lifted skyward. When it gained some altitude she began to circle, the bells on her legs tinkling faintly in the air above us. No one said a word.

Higher and higher she gyrated toward the gray dome of clouds above us. Everyone followed her with their eyes, murmuring as she found the circling thermal. Suddenly the dog let out a series of yelps and pointed, his tail straight out behind him, his front paw tucked underneath his chest. The hawk was now almost out of sight, only a speck circling far up in the sky. Then, like an utterance from some archaic language, the Count shouted "Hie! Hie! Hie!" and the dog, ravenous with his cue to flush the birds, barked and leapt into the bushes. In a second, as if they were part of their own death plan, a covey of grouse exploded out of the underbrush, all in different directions, calling and flapping their wings in terror, trying to find one another, trying to flee what they thought was the predator. But they hadn't a clue.

The Count's falcon stooped straight toward the Earth like a missile, faster than any living creature. Locked into the site of the flush, and in a perfect bullet shape, she descended, wings tucked, her keen eyes on one thing only. In one ecstatic instant the life of a grouse ended in a cloud of feathers, its down wafting earthward like an afterthought.

Everyone applauded and cheered. The dogs yelped, drowning out any human voice. The falconer ran to his bird, offering it fresh meat in exchange for the cleanly killed grouse, first of the brace to be served later for dinner. Trey's eyes shone; clearly, he was both agitated and excited by the kill.

At first, I was speechless, but then I couldn't help myself. "That was awful. And beautiful, yes, yes, the choreography—but it's—it's dreadful, too, isn't it?" I was still back in the copse with the grouse who'd been totally taken by surprise. Though I caught fish to eat, I wasn't prepared for the tactics of this ambush, the enlistment of other creatures to bag a man's quarry, or the bloodthirsty baying of the dogs. And all those feathers.

"Bollocks, Christine. You just don't get it, do you?" Trey said. "In actual fact, you are *defiling* the moment. A *perfect* moment, no less." The Count glanced over at us, startled and questioning. Trey strode off, his long arms swinging, leaving me alone with the women who politely turned away from my humiliation. I blinked back tears. The Count's falcon ripped apart the hunk of fresh meat and devoured it in huge gulps, blood dribbling down her breast.

Chapter 9.

Issues

IN THE COLD ARENA OUR breath puffs out in small clouds. Ken wraps his bare hands around a steaming cup of coffee. "If you can actually *see* what your horse is thinking, you can help him find his way," Ken says, addressing a woman on a sorrel mustang. The horse fidgets in the line of six horses and riders. "We need to read them constantly. Watch their eyes, their bodies. See where their attention is. And if *we* pay attention, that horse's story will reveal itself to us. It will tell us loud and clear what might have gone wrong in the past."

Next to Buddy and me, my friend Stephanie sits smartly on her huge Friesian, Mateo. Over sixteen hands high, Mateo looks like a medieval war horse. His hoofs are the size of salad plates, and his mane and tail are jet black, bushy, and full. Stephanie's face is tense today. Recently, when the stable owner led Mateo from his stall to the turn-out paddock, he had swung his huge hind-end to kick him all the way across the driveway, ten feet or more. If he'd struck his head, the man would be dead. As it was, he'd gone to the hospital with several broken ribs.

Mateo swishes his tail. Stephanie carefully backs him up out of the line of horses. An excellent horsewoman, she rides beautifully and is always looking to learn more. She's even hauled Mateo to

Arizona to attend a week-long clinic at the ranch of a well-known trainer.

Though mesmerized by Mateo's beauty, I am always careful when riding with Stephanie to move Buddy into the lead so as not to be anywhere near Mateo's hindquarters. Next to Mateo, Buddy looks like a Lilliputian from Gulliver's travels.

My admiration for Stephanie does not stop at her riding skills. She is honest about Mateo's problems. Where many horse owners might mask the difficulties—either by pretending they didn't exist or by blaming the horse—Stephanie keeps looking for solutions. She'd bought him as a yearling, sight unseen, and when the driver arrived from several states away, he unloaded the colt in a hurry and said, "This horse has issues. You better watch out," then left without another word.

In the five years she'd owned him, Stephanie has single-handedly doctored him through a bad horse fight where he'd been kicked in the cannon bone. She'd researched all sorts of ways to make him physically and mentally sounder. And she found Ken. She's kept at it, too, even though her horse is becoming more difficult. The previous week he'd bolted when Stephanie was riding him down a busy road. She was pitched off and landed on the pavement, glad she was wearing her helmet.

After that, Ken recommended she get a stronger bit for safety, even though all of us were aiming toward a light bit and a loose rein. Stephanie mucked Mateo's stall, fed him, brushed him till he shone, and gave this magnificent beast every luxury she could afford. But sometimes he had a cold look to his eye. I felt for her. I knew what it was to love someone whose eyes could change from soft to hard in an instant. I knew the heartbreak of thinking *this time it will be different.*

Chapter 10.

❧ *Adrift* ❧

ANY WOMAN WHO HAS LOST a hoped-for pregnancy knows how deep the desire is to replace it—like, right away. It's tempting for people to say (and a couple friends did), "It wasn't a person yet; you didn't even know him. You will have another." But for those of us who really *did* know that spark of life inside, such comments can be hurtful, as if what you'd experienced was not actually real. How can one explain the irrational but primal need to replace what was lost, whatever the cost? For me this relationship felt like a moral imperative—to make things *good* or *better*. In a strange way, losing the child had made me more fearful of losing other things, including Trey, even with his outbursts which, with the help of Lewis, were becoming rare. My body was crying to have that baby back; it just couldn't stand the empty space.

And, if one does get pregnant again—as I did that spring with great surprise—you actually feel vindicated: All is right with the world after all! See? What was lost is now found! The story has a happy ending!

Spring in Riojos was dreamy, literally. Trey and I were careful with each other and both cautiously excited about the baby. I slept constantly, drugged by hormones and the high desert air. In early April we even took a two-week trip to Tobago, where a friend of mine had invited us to team-lead a writing workshop about birds. Travel expenses were included in the stipend. I'd worried the trip might endanger the baby, but the doctor was encouraging, so we went ahead. "It will be good for all of us," Trey said, laying his hand on my belly. And he was right. The teaching was light, and much of the time we sipped mango smoothies while flocks of wild parrots chortled and swooped over our heads. We celebrated Trey's birthday there, too, and he adored the present I found for him, made by an artisan on the island: a small, round wooden box with a pair of carved parrots as the handle, their lime-green wings outstretched, their beaks just touching.

"That's us!" Trey said. The Caribbean light gave his olive skin a rich glow.

Once back in New Mexico, rested and the baby growing, Trey and I settled into the calm rhythms of Rocking H life. We saw Lewis weekly, and he helped us reach yet another "weir." The high desert bloomed, and Trey made a guest list for our wedding and shopped for steak and crates of San Pellegrino water. On Saturdays Trey loved going to yard sales, and one morning he proudly returned with a green plastic child's wading pool. "Can't you just see our little fellow splashing in this?" That same week we witnessed our baby's heartbeat on the ultrasound. The screen showed a rhythmic little blob. "Well, there's our Joey!" Trey said, grinning like a kid himself.

This time I had named the baby. The little offspring stuffed in a kangaroo's pouch seemed less ostentatious than a Greek god. Surely such a gentle name would keep him well below the radar of capricious gods.

No such luck. A month after returning from the Caribbean and well into my second trimester, I miscarried again, and this time I literally took to my bed. For days and days. I could not face the world; all I wanted was to sleep. My friend Belinda warned me that the Percocet prescribed for pain was terribly habit-forming, so I stopped that immediately, but if anyone were to say, "Hey! How are you?!" I wanted to run away. Who can really reply, "Well, just great! I had a baby, but now I don't"? I avoided the INFANTS aisle in Walmart with its soft blankets, snugglies, and tiny overalls. I stopped shopping for groceries so I wouldn't have to see anyone. And when my spirits didn't seem to bounce back, Mom and Rosemary came down with Celia for a week of family fortification. The timing couldn't have been better. Trey was in Dallas selling some of the books from the Santa Fe collection, and we spent our days peacefully making meals with Sas, and Mom read in the hammock under the locust tree, while baby Celia delighted in the cats. It felt so good to be able to talk about my sorrow, to receive their help and tenderness, to stand on familiar, solid ground.

What makes miscarriage particularly devastating, after all, is its secrecy. If my babies had been born and died, sympathy notes would have appeared in my mailbox. Friends would have brought casseroles. Besides my family and a few close friends, I'd kept it quiet for good reason. And I couldn't tell those people now, as they would then have to rewind, imagine me pregnant, and then fast-forward to the grisly details. I'd have to comfort *them*.

In addition to mourning, shame seems to accompany this kind of death. "A bad egg," the hospital doctor had told me before my D & C. "A bad egg!?" To the physician I was a medical backfire, but I wanted to wail, "It was my child! I saw his heart beating!! He had a name!" All my body's functions had been charging full speed ahead, every cell protecting what was inside of me, and suddenly the train had screeched to a halt, my body asking, "Now what?"

By the fall, I was still treading water, unsure how to proceed. I'd been seeing a fertility doctor, but the whole process seemed utterly antithetical to my idea of motherhood or how one creates a family.

So I called my mother.

"Oh, honey, I'll come right back down there if that would help." It had only been a month since she, Rosemary, and Celia had been at the Rocking H.

"Oh, Mom…," I said, moved by her unsolicited offer. "I'm just tired of being sad, that's all," I said. But then a strange pause filled the other end of the line. "Are you there, Mom?"

"Oh, yes," she said. "And I really can come down again. It's no trouble." She laughed. "I still haven't unpacked my travel bag!"

When Mom, Rosemary, and Celia had left the month before, I had waved goodbye tearfully, wishing I could return with them, back to the moist, comforting green of my childhood. When they disappeared down the road, I turned back to the Rocking H alone, dust blowing across the mesa.

Mom continued on the phone, "Remember, now: Your life is filled with creativity, and you always get the things that you long for. You have so many amazing friends and amazing work, big adventures. Even if it might not be in the plan to have a baby, things will work out for you. In fact, knowing you, you'll *make* them work out!" She laughed.

I breathed a sigh of relief and laughed, too. "How is it that when I talk to you things never seem as bad?"

"Oh, just sit at my feet…," she said with her usual irony. Mom always had a knack for giving comfort without sentimentality. When we were kids, if one of us was home from school with the flu, she'd say, "Let's just plump you up with these nice fresh pillows, shall we?" Then she'd tuck us into bed and read aloud from *The Secret Garden* or *Just So Stories*. When it was clear we were no longer sick, however, she'd say briskly, "Get up!" even if we tried to force a loud cough or beg one more chapter out of her. No go. No wallowing.

In that phone call with Mom, however, I failed to tell her about another worry I'd been nursing since she'd been in Riojos. Trey had begun to spend more and more time with a falconry friend in Santa Fe. At first he said he was doing some book sales, but sometimes he didn't come back until nearly midnight, and he finally admitted he was helping a friend with his hawk. And then little things irritated him more than ever. A poor Internet connection, a news profile about a politician's infidelities, or something as small as Callie pooping outside the cat box.

But then he'd click back (often exhausted, as if he'd been ill with a fever) into his fun-loving self.

"Look!" he said one night after bursting home from a visit to an Albuquerque used bookstore. "Look what I found—isn't it fantastic?" He unrolled a large, nineteenth-century print onto the dining room table. The picture he unveiled at first appeared to be a benign Victorian domestic scene: A well-dressed man reclines on an ornate settee. A dog snoozes on the Persian rug. A drawing room perhaps? At the center of the picture plane, perched on the man's gauntlet-clad arm, is a hooded falcon.

I burst out laughing. We both were amused at the besotted man staring at his hawk in rapture. "I couldn't help but buy it." Trey laughed again. "The dealer was reluctant to let it go, but I gave him a fair price," he said. When I leaned closer, however, the most arresting part of the print was not the hawk; it was the figure of a young wife in the background, tentatively looking through a doorway, as if she'd just discovered her beloved with his mistress. The ribbons in her hair hang limp, her body is in shadow, her face downcast. In stylish script below the scene the title reads, "The Heart's Misgivings."

"The Heart's Misgivings?" I said aloud, "Well!" And we both laughed again with abandon, back in the shared Land of Us. Oh, how I loved to hear Trey laugh like that.

Eventually, though, he began disappearing for longer periods. Suddenly his old friend Blane—whom I'd never met—would need his help, and he'd be off for the day with Blane and his hawks. He'd return with a distracted smile, waving off any concerns I might have, though it got difficult to ask him about what was actually happening. He'd talk seriously about "trust," and I retreated in my own thoughts, feeling too claustrophobic to rally, actually relieved he was gone. Plus, when he brought up "trust," it reminded me of some dive of a restaurant that advertises "Good Food!"

And then, something even more confusing: the more quiet and introspective I became, the more he craved me, like a bird of prey going straight for exposed blood. His lovemaking grew needy and ravenous, as if he feared I was going to disappear. He'd even given me gold falconry-bell earrings for my birthday "So you can never get lost. Never get away from me," he said, squeezing his long arm around me and pressing his hard lips into my scalp.

All of this I kept from my mother, who had her own difficulties to deal with. Her memory was clearly diminishing. One night on the phone she laughed and said, "Sometimes I can't even remember my old recipe for poaching fish!" as if such a thing were a mere bug bite. Neither Dad, Paul, Rosemary, nor I could believe that Mom—of all people—would have problems in this department. She was the memory vault for the whole family. And, though she'd seemed tired (and yes, a little forgetful) when she was in Riojos, swinging in the hammock with Badger, I hadn't wanted to see any failings in my mother, especially since I was trying to sort out my own life.

She'd always handled the books for Dad's travel marketing business in addition to their own personal finances. A month before she came to Riojos, she'd accidentally deleted all the QuickBooks files, leaving an arid vista on the hard drive. She'd reluctantly turned over the finances to an accountant. But I still could not picture Mom wandering around not remembering things. She knew every one of her children's friends' names from kindergarten on, the variety of finch at the feeder, and the intricacies of my father's budget. Not to mention the authors of the zillions of books she'd read. Plus, she hated the mess of unsavory conditions, and this memory disorder was not her kind of thing at all.

Now I asked if she'd had the Alzheimer's test. Dad had told me he'd set one up for her, but I hadn't heard anything since.

"What good will it do me?" Mom said, another pause on the line stretching out a beat too long. "Knowing if I have it? There's nothing to be done about it anyway. There's no cure." She sighed. "So I find out I have it? What then?" She said she'd decided not to take the final diagnostic test. *What?* I thought. *Mom, the advocate of Knowledge is Power?* This was strange news indeed. I recalled the lapses she'd had recently, especially when a lot of information was coming at her. Odd silences, like the ones on the phone, where I wasn't sure if she was bored, or if the connection had faltered.

"Adrift. That's the word," Mom said. "I feel adrift." Mom was never one to whine about health issues. When she'd had breast cancer in her early fifties and sustained radiation burns around her lymph nodes under her arms, she said, after the doctor had marveled at her outcome and recovery, "Well, at least I won't ever have to shave or wear deodorant again!"

"We'll see how it works out," she said cheerfully. "But I've decided that I'm not going to ruin this stage of my life agonizing about it." She was quiet for a moment. "What a waste to spend time worrying, so I'm going to enjoy this time the best I can." I pictured her on her deck with her pots of herbs and flowers, a vestige of her former bucolic life in Meadowdale. "It's the same for you, Christine. Enjoy this time of your life. Just let it unfold." She reminded me of the time when we were first searching for a horse and I'd been so disappointed when someone else had bought the horse I had my heart set on. But then we got Lightfoot, who became the love of my life. Mom's voice came through the phone like clear water. "You thought that chestnut mare was the only horse for you, remember?"

Chapter 11.

⟻Trust⟻

KEN RUBS HIS GLOVELESS HANDS together and blows on them. A woman in a huge parka brings him another cup of coffee.

"Used incorrectly, a bit can be torture for a horse." Ken walks over to Buddy's head, pauses, looks up at me, and then lays his hand on Buddy's cheek. "But with the right hands, a horse can get over discomfort with the bit. There are ways to help a horse find relaxation in his jaw and ultimately softness in his whole body." Ken takes hold of my right rein as if he were the rider.

"See?" he says, making sure everyone has a view of his hand. "I'm just holding this rein with as much pressure as I would a dance partner. He touches my knee to illustrate how little pressure he was using on the rein. "Just the tiniest contact. Add contact by the ounce until you feel the horse give you a response, then release, so he knows that it's the right and easy thing."

Buddy doesn't give. He braces his head and even from up on his back I can feel his grumpiness.

"What we're looking for, really, is the response," Ken says. "Which may be bracing, as Buddy's doing now. But that's actually an indication that he *cares* about this, about you. It's not indifference. You *matter* to him." I try to hide my smile.

As Ken talks, his hand on the rein remains soft and clear. No changing the pressure, no pulling or yanking. Just a steady, light reminder to Buddy to give slightly in his jaw.

"Until you get his response, you wait. You just wait. And listen. Until the horse offers even the tiniest give." Ken's hand moves with Buddy's head as Buddy pushes his jaw against the soft pressure. Then, as if a window opens, Buddy's jaw relaxes, his eyes soften, and Ken releases the rein.

"There! Did you see that?" Ken's eyes light up as if he'd spotted a rare bird. Buddy's ears went forward when he felt the release, the quiet. I'd felt it, too. But getting the timing of the release was so hard. It took all my concentration to try to wrap my mind around what Ken was trying to show me there in the cold arena. It was so subtle, deceptively simple, and yet so difficult.

The books I'd been devouring about horsemanship showed me that "Natural Horsemanship" (as it is currently branded by big-name clinicians) isn't new at all. In fact, it has roots back in Classical Greece. I had run across a treatise written in 350 B.C. by the historian Xenophon. He outlined the same horsemanship philosophy about softness and partnership. In fact, according to Xenophon, a well-trained cavalryman's horse was often worth more than his own house. In medieval as well as Greek times, horses were trained for war, not the show ring. Those Andalusians and huge Lipizzaners charged, piaffed, and leapt like dancers. But the best ones were not pummeled into obedience. Nor were they taught to do such supple maneuvers by harsh bits and tie-downs that kept their heads from tossing. A soldier needed a horse who would go into battle eagerly and athletically—as an honest and willing partner.

Yes, there were horsemen who whacked their horses into submission and castrated the stallions in order to have a modicum of control, but one book by a contemporary European horseman says there was a special sect of knights in medieval Europe, a monastic order, who held the secret to victory in battle. These Knights Templar apparently won their battles because they only fought the human enemy. Not their horses. They had learned the quiet language of the equine herd, the same thing Ken was teaching. The knights worked with their horses slowly and carefully, never ever using punishment. The best horsemen possessed the kind of personal strength found in lead mares or stallions. Monks were carefully vetted to join this sect, and apparently, even today in Spain and France, they speak of it not as "high school," a common dressage term for highly trained horses, but the "monastic school."

With the medieval horses' trust in these monk-knights, anything was possible. A color reproduction of a thirteenth-century French fresco depicts knights riding in full armor, and the horses wear no bits or bridles at all. The warriors brandish a shield in one hand and a sword in another, subtle cues obviously coming only from the seat and legs. The knights had another thing going for them, too. If they did happen to fall to the ground during battle (the weight of armor must have been enormous), they were never abandoned by their mounts. The secret and powerful relationship with their horses literally saved their lives.

"The bit itself doesn't really matter, ultimately," Ken tells us, standing in front of the line of horses and riders. "Well, that's not entirely true—but the *kind* of bit isn't the issue. Some kind of trauma happened with Buddy around the bit, as it has in most horses, and we need to show him that it doesn't have to be painful, physically or mentally. In fact, it will eventually become a comfortable place for him, a more finely tuned connection to you." Buddy's ears swivel back when Ken places a tiny bit of pressure on his mouth with the rein.

He laughs at Buddy's black lips twitching slightly, and his eyes that seem to be saying, "Geesh!"

"This horse doesn't hide how he feels, does he?" We all laugh, Buddy's thoughts so clearly visible on his face. "Actually, this is good." Ken glances up at me. "I like to see a horse having an honest opinion. It means he isn't dead to the world, he's not buried under all the layers of resistance or numb submission. Buddy may have a little history as we all do, but he is not damaged goods. He's got a strong sense of who he is." Buddy's ears perk forward.

"Have you seen those English dressage horses all strapped up in equipment to keep their heads set?" Ken shakes his head. "Their riders' arms ropey and sinewy from pulling on the reins? Making them do maneuvers that horses can do naturally without apparatus?" He scrunches his Australian hat down tighter on his thick, gray hair. "That is not dressage as it was originally practiced. Masterful dressage riders often take a whole year just to perfect the horse's walk, so the horse can learn to carry the rider's weight in perfect balance. We don't need equipment to do that. We just need time and patience."

Ken taps a menthol smoke out of the wrinkled pack. "Most of those horses in the show ring are not willing horses. Just look at their eyes…filled with discomfort, fear, resignation, and no small amount of anger."

I remember an earlier conversation I'd had with Ken about Stephanie's Mateo. Her horse had kicked her again, against the pipe fence. Ken said he worried about her safety, even after he'd worked with Mateo at his own farm. When he finished the month of training, Ken had discussed with Stephanie the option of putting him down. "Each time I send a horse like that back to its owner, I think about where the holes are," he'd said. "I lie awake at night going over it in my mind."

Next to me, Stephanie calmly backs Mateo up from the line of horses again, his tail swishing. Ken goes on to explain to the group, "The most dangerous horses are those who have been spoiled or mistreated. If that's not dealt with, it will always appear at unexpected times." I know Stephanie has not mistreated Mateo, but who knows what had happened before he came to her?

"Many horses adapt, even if they've been traumatized," Ken says. "They can learn to behave on a surface level. I mean—they learn to say, 'Okay, I can put a bit in my mouth. Okay, I will tolerate you getting on my back with that saddle. Okay, I can change leads.' And they do it. It's easier to shut down. But if a horseman or woman actually gets who they are, sees where the trouble is, and offers a better deal—some horses can't handle the honesty. Often such powerful recognition is just too much for a damaged horse to take. They hold it together for a long time, until wham!—they pop a cork. The past just comes rushing back."

Chapter 12.

∽Unhinged∽

Trey's Trooper lurched into the driveway. He hopped out and opened the back door. A hooded hawk sat on a perch on the seat. It ruffled its feathers, and its head swiveled to catch our voices.

"Wow, Trey...," I said, setting down the basket of lettuce from the garden. I stared at the bird in disbelief.

"It's okay," Trey said. "I'm just helping Blane." He lifted the falcon off the perch and grabbed a bag. "His wife made it clear." Then he broke into a strange hollow laugh. "She told him, 'Either the hawk goes, or I go!' But really. This is okay, seriously. I'm doing Blane a favor. Lisa is a great girl. I've seen her fly." (Lisa?) The hawk now sat on Trey's gloved wrist like a ship's masthead, regal and cold.

I tried to welcome Lisa into the family, but the cats were terrified of her (even with the hood). I half-heartedly justified Trey's decision by thinking he needed something after the blow of losing another hoped-for child. But he hadn't asked me, and I was baffled as to what he was trying to prove with Lisa. While I worked at my desk, Trey strode around the ranch with a new mission, Lisa bravely on his arm. One morning I came out with my coffee to find the green wading pool he'd bought for Joey smack in the center of the patio. The fresh water glinted as Trey lowered Lisa in to bathe.

That week Lisa went everywhere with us. The diaper bag with Lisa's meat and water dish came, too, even when we went shopping. I told myself it was the same as Badger, who had accompanied me on my outings when I lived in Boston. He'd ridden on my shoulder all over town, pre-9/11 he'd flown in a carry-on under my airline seat and accompanied me to teach my classes. I'd even taken him in a basket to my part-time evening paralegal job at the corporate law offices in Boston. Wasn't Lisa the same as my beloved cat? Couldn't I just embrace her in the spirit of animal delight? Was I the crazy one? I was so confused it was hard to tell.

One night Trey wore his falconry gauntlet to a dinner party—Lisa perched on his forearm—until she got situated on the back of a chair, her head swiveling as she listened to conversation beneath her dark leather hood. People were charmed by Trey's sidekick, welcoming raptor and Trey as if they were royalty. Another dinner guest cooed, flashing her eyes at Trey, "I think it's—like—sooooooooo exotic!" and touched Lisa's hood with a bright red fingernail.

When a shipment of dead baby chicks arrived by UPS, both Sas and I agreed that the Rocking H was taking a turn (or stoop). Trey wanted to store the chicks in my refrigerator, but I drew the line and he marched to his own studio. The next day live pigeons appeared in the tool shed. "They are for training," Trey told me in a voice filled with the authority of a professor, adding that the door must remain closed at all times and *no one* should enter the Pigeon House. "We train hawks to kill pigeons first, then grouse," he said, setting down his glass of iced tea on the counter with an emphatic clink. The pigeons' nervous coos wafted through the open window.

Very soon our landlord, Arnold, began to fret about the hawk and its paraphernalia. Trey immediately became incensed. "Arnold does not realize that I have rights here!" Trey said, as he strode into my casita and loomed over my desk. "And I'm getting everything in writing." He waved a stack of papers toward my face, then slapped one sheet down and signed it with a flourish. "Here. You witnessed this. Read it!" he said, pushing it back in my face. The letter, addressed to our landlord (who lived a mere hundred feet away), accused Arnold of a flawed character, even suggesting that his earlier bout with throat cancer was a result of selfishness.

"Oh, no nooooo...," I said, handing the letter back to Trey as if it were poisoned. "You cannot send this to Arnold. He is our friend. He's done so much for us here. And he's uncomfortable with Lisa. Maybe if you just had a conversation with him?...instead of all these letters..."

"No. We need to document every bit of this," he said and left the house. The wind kicked up, and fallen locust tree leaves whirled in a mini dust devil on the patio.

When the Arnold letters were revealed, it became clear that this wasn't about Lisa—or even falconry. It was about Trey. The question was, was he suffering some emotional breakdown because he was incapable of addressing his partner's grief? My mind immediately gravitated to the sanity of Lewis's office; Trey and I had an appointment for the following Monday, but I told him he needed to stay in his own casita until he was calmer, in a less contentious state of mind. Almost as if he hadn't heard me, he marched right to the vegetable garden carrying a twenty-pound hammer from my toolbox with which he smashed the frame he'd built for his compost heap. With each strike, he dislodged another wooden slat that flew into the kale, destroying our Eden in just a few blows. He finally threw down the hammer and strode away, leaving the compost heap looking like a pile of corpses.

I'd made plans to attend my college reunion in Oregon that weekend, and I felt both relieved and scared to leave. Our Monday appointment with Lewis was a beacon in the distance. The next night, when I arrived at my friend Dan's apartment after an alumni dinner, he met me at the door. "Come in and sit down," he said. "I'm going to pour you a drink." My delight was doused by the look on his face. "Trey called," he said.

"What? He called here?" My first fear was that something had happened to Badger or Callie. I'd specifically appointed Sas to look after them.

Dan set a glass of bourbon on the table. "Apparently your land-lord—um—has ordered Trey to leave the Rocking H Ranch."

I sat down with a thump. I'd planned to tell Dan and his girl-friend, Helen, about the Trey situation the next day, but I'd so wanted my reunion to be free of the complications of Riojos. The news washed over me with dread.

"Your landlord sent him a certified letter," Dan said and took a sip of his drink, the ice cubes clinking. "But I guess the letter was for him, not you. According to Trey, he must leave by the end of the month."

My bourbon sat sweating, untouched.

"He sounded—how shall I say it?—*unhinged*," Dan said diplomatically.

Shaken and embarrassed by this unsavory news, I cut my reunion short and flew home early the next morning, driving the three hours from the airport to the Rocking H. Trey obviously hadn't shaved since I'd banished him from my bed and casita. His eyes were empty and cold. There was dirt under his fingernails, and his clothes looked as if he'd slept in them. Baby chick feathers lay on the floor, and Lisa sat on the back of the chair, the top-knot on her hood bouncing with each cock of her head. His house smelled like death.

"Hi, Trey," I said quietly, standing in the open door. He looked up with a vacant stare. "Tell me about Arnold. What's happening exactly?"

"You don't understand," Trey said, rearranging a pile of papers on the table. He looked right at me, as if he'd finally found the words I needed to hear. "You have to get this straight right now: being with a falconer is like being with a doctor."

A doctor? I started to smile, thinking he was joking. But he leapt to the next sentence like a racehorse leaving the gate.

"It's a constant job, you see. I must always be on call." I pictured him with a stethoscope. But Trey's unwashed hair made him look old and sinister. His mouth, so charming when turned up in his radiant smile, had caved in, and his lips nearly disappeared in the shadow of his face. Was I somehow complicit in his descent into this altered reality? Where was that man who knew the names of my childhood animals? The one who had made love to me so deeply and gently our bodies could not get enough?

Trey then touched each finger to its opposite finger on the other hand in a prayerful tableau and took a breath, as if beginning a long speech. "It's perfectly clear now that you're not on my side."

"Your side? When did this become about sides?" I breathed in and held it.

"You didn't stand up to Arnold and his accusations," Trey said. "You just left town. Without a thought about me." I glanced around the room at the dead chicks, the scale to measure their weight, hawk poop on the floor, books and papers strewn about. "My documentation proves it all." Trey straightened a pile of notebooks on the table, and one fell on the floor. Lisa jumped.

"I'll see you tomorrow then?" I said, backing slowly toward the door. "At our meeting with Lewis? Shall we go together?" After all my hope, I couldn't imagine what Lewis could do now, but it seemed important for me to have a witness besides Sas.

"I'll meet you there," Trey said and stood up, his eyes pitiless, like Lisa's. I turned and stepped outside. Puffs of chick down lifted as I shut the door.

Chapter 13.

Choices

STEPHANIE ARRIVES AT MY DOORSTEP, and her face tells me things are not good. She begins to cry. "Come in," I say, ushering her into the living room. "What is it?" I ask, hugging her immediately. Her sobs throb against my chest.

"Mateo's done it again," she says, pulling away. Her hands shake, and she looks pale. "I was leading him—usually I have my eye out. But this time it seemed really premeditated. Like he was aiming right at me." She breaks down again. "And when I finally let go of the lead rope—there's no holding that horse back—he twirled around and both back legs shot out in unison, right at me. *At me.*" Stephanie takes a clean tissue out of her pocket and blows her nose. "If I'd been in the line of fire, I would not be here right now." I picture Mateo's impossibly huge hoofs.

"What are you going to do?" I ask, dreading the answer.

She glances out the living room window. "Well, I can't sell him. Who will take him? Who knows what he might do to somebody else…" Her eyes are bloodshot from days of agonizing. "And even if I did sell him…How do I know that person wouldn't abuse him? Do terrible things to *him?*" Stephanie takes her car keys out of her pocket. "He has moments of real sweetness." She closes her eyes. "He really does. He just can't hold onto them when he needs to.

And when *I* need him to. Only once have I walked up the path that he hasn't come all the way across the paddock to greet me at the gate, often at a lovely canter." Her hands tremble. "I've always believed that I was the only person Mateo could feel safe with. His home was with me. And now...?" she pauses, her eyes wet with tears. "I can't be safe with him."

Chapter 14.

❧ *The Bridge* ❧

WHEN I PULLED INTO LEWIS'S office, the outline of Riojos Mountain looked like a painting, its blue shadows velvety and thick, a luminosity that most painters fail to capture, no matter how hard they try.

Lewis immediately read my stricken face. "I'm scared, Lewis," I said but had little time to explain—or even mention how, that morning, I'd discovered my birthday present to Trey crushed to pieces on my porch, the parrots' wings broken off and the rest of the box scattered in splinters. Just as I sat down to give Lewis a few details, Trey burst in the door. He wore a sport coat, clean khakis, and dress loafers. He had showered and shaved, and he carried a leather briefcase which, oddly, made him look like a lawyer.

"Hello, Lewis," Trey said, dropping a public health brochure titled ANGER into my lap before taking a seat.

"Hello, Trey," Lewis said.

Trey settled in, hugging his briefcase. Despite the tension in the room, Lewis relaxed into his chair, his pencil poised.

"So. What seems to be going on now? I see that you two arrived separately. What's happened since we last met?"

Trey sat straight and tall. He filled the chair. "Well, Lewis, there is a lot to report." He immediately launched into the details of

Arnold's demand that he leave the Rocking H, stopping only to reach into his breast pocket to retrieve the folded certified letter.

Lewis nodded, "Did it occur to you that any of this might make Christine uncomfortable?"

The hollow, false laugh, Trey's intake of breath labored.

"Now why are you laughing exactly?" Lewis said, truly bewildered.

"Well, it's just that she's really not the one to be talking about discomfort. She is the one making *me* uncomfortable."

"And how is that?" Lewis tipped his head.

"First of all, I'm only interested in the truth here, Lewis. What's right and wrong." He popped the latches on his briefcase and pulled out one of several spiral-bound notebooks. "It's Christine's fault that I have to leave the Rocking H." He flipped through the pages. "If you will allow me here, Lewis, I have evidence. I've recorded everything in these notebooks. You'll see." He began reading aloud from his own journal entries, as if he were a commentator on the BBC. He looked up at Lewis for affirmation as Arnold's registered letter reentered the story. When Lewis remained quiet, Trey hesitated, then launched back into a cross-referenced section in Notebook #2.

Finally, Lewis held up his hand. "I get the picture, Trey." He took a breath, quickly recalibrating his approach. Clearly, he had never seen Trey behave this way in his one-on-one meetings.

Trey laid the open notebooks on his lap. Lewis took another slow breath and turned to me, then over to Trey. "So Christine tells me she's been feeling scared, Trey. Not from the hawk itself, but how it's affected your relationship."

"Lisa," Trey said. "The hawk's name is Lisa."

"Lisa, then," Lewis said. "What can you say about this, Trey?

Trey pushed his glasses up his nose. "I'm the one who should be scared. She's so emotional these days, I just can't predict what she's going to do. Ever since the last miscarriage, she's gone off the deep end. And, to be honest, I'm worried for Lisa. I don't think she's safe with Christine around. Or Sas or Arnold. It's probably good I'm leaving the ranch. Lisa would be in grave danger now."

"Grave danger?" Lewis's eyes flickered with mild alarm.

"Lewis, don't you get it?" Trey leaned full torso toward Lewis's chair, "You, of all people?" The sudden physicality of Trey prompted Lewis to take a slow, quiet breath. Trey sat back and folded his hands, and a smile began to form on his lips as if he were the therapist treating a very sick patient. "It's just that Christine is not facing her fears, Lewis," he said confidentially. "Or her anger. She has so much anger in there." He pointed at me without looking my way. "But the most important detail here?" Trey crossed his legs. "It's bloody obvious: She did not support me, her husband-to-be. In actual fact, she betrayed me. And I do not tolerate betrayal, Lewis. Frankly? I'm glad I didn't marry her."

Something clean and primal surged through my body, the same impulse that drives a fisherman from a falling boulder, flushes a grouse from a baying dog, provokes a horse to bolt. Without thinking, my body rose and carried me right out of that chair, right out the door. The sunset on Riojos Mountain had long faded, and the October sky was now a glass bowl of stars in which the constellations were shifting.

After getting home, I turned out all the lights, shoved the kitchen table against the door, and called Sas. She was packing to leave for Berkeley. Her boyfriend, John, was sick, and she was eager to tend to him. She'd been waiting for my return from the therapy session but hadn't expected me so soon.

"Are you okay?" she asked. "Where's Trey? Did you go in separate cars?"

"I'm leaving," I told her.

"Leaving? Like leaving? Leaving *town*?"

"Yes," I said. "I'm going home. Tomorrow morning. Can you come over? Say goodbye?"

I let her in the back door, and we lit a fire in my fireplace, the first—and last—of the season. Sweet piñon smoke rose up the chimney, its fragrance one of the many things I dreaded leaving behind. I recounted the session with Lewis, how it appeared that Trey had had some kind of a break (or was this who he really was?). I told her how I'd left right in the middle of the session. "Trey's still there with Lewis," I said. "Or not. I don't know."

"Wow," Sas said. "Wow. What can I do to help you leave?"

My eyes smarted with tears. "I'm just going to take a few things, lock up, and go," I said. "I'm just glad you're leaving, too." Neither of us felt safe around Trey now, and the thought of my dear friend living next to him seemed downright hellish. How could our life here in Riojos have exploded so quickly? Where had our bucolic idyll gone? I flashed back to an evening with Sas several years earlier—long before Trey—when I'd lived alone on the Rio Rondo. I'd caught two trout for dinner and had invited Sas to share them with me. It was one of those Riojos evenings where the light was ambrosial, the air clear and mesmerizing. When Sas saw the trout I'd caught and cleaned for us, she said, "Oh, I've got to take a picture." We arranged the fish on one of my red plates and put it down in the grass by the river.

"This is it," Sas had said. "This is life. Right now. There isn't anything else. The beauty. These fish."

Now, standing in the dark there with my best friend, preparing to leave the life I'd created out of nothing, I was painfully aware that *this* was life, too. How could I reconcile it except to say *This is always It. Even* this?

Finally, I hugged Sas tight, and we agreed that we'd talk once she was back in Berkeley. "You'd better leave early," she said, giving me another squeeze.

Before Sas closed the door quietly behind her, she turned back. The firelight flickered shadows on the huge exposed log beams.

"You're doing the right thing. Really." She disappeared into the night, and I lodged another chair against the back door. I looked around to see what few things I could fit into my tiny Ford Festiva. As I was zipping my laptop into its case, the phone rang, and my heart jumped. Hands trembling, I picked it up.

"Are you all right?" A familiar voice met my ear.

"Oh, Lewis," I said, sighing with relief. "I'm so glad it's you. But I need to leave town. I'm driving home. Tomorrow morning. To my family. In Washington State…" I held back a sob, then breathed in and told the truth for the first time out loud: "If I stay here I will die. Spiritually, if not physically." How could I admit to Lewis how much I had loved Trey? And did even now—though I never wanted to lay eyes upon him again. Ever.

"I support you completely," my therapist said. This came as a relief. "And you do know, don't you, that you couldn't have done a thing to prevent what happened with Trey?" He stopped, as if sorting out his thoughts. "It's his own choice," he said. "He had such a chance at something big—with you and his new life here—that he could have released himself from his past. But ultimately—at least for now—he just wasn't up to the task. He could go only so far. He stretched and stretched—admirably so—but then he snapped." I didn't know what to say.

"Oh, and one more thing," Lewis said. I wondered if he was going to tell me what had happened after I'd blown out of his office, leaving him alone with Trey. "Are your doors locked?" Not only were the doors dead-bolted, I'd had the locks changed before I'd gone to Oregon. I told him so. "If he does come to your place, do not engage with him. Call me and 911 immediately if you need to." I thanked him, but it was devastating to witness the needle on my heart's compass spin 180 degrees away from Trey. My home was no longer here.

After hanging up with Lewis, I put an extra chair against the kitchen door. Trey had never hurt me physically, but I wasn't taking any chances. I looked around at my dark, little house. With sudden resolve, I began packing: two cat carriers, two fishing rods, two flutes, a new translation of the Book of Psalms, the collected works of Theodore Roethke, Denise Levertov's last book, a few clothes in a duffel, a printer, and a small box of bills and bank statements. I stacked it all by the back door, ready to load in the morning.

Before turning out my bedside lamp, I paused to look at one of my favorite pieces by Sas, which hung by my bed. She'd made it especially for me when we'd first met: a three-dimensional collage, housed in a dictionary-size Plexiglas box. The background was thickly painted with umber, pink, and gold acrylic. She'd glued a dried snakeskin to the painting's surface, too. Barely visible under more layers of paint, a naked Adam and Eve smiled at the huge leering serpent coiling up a tree. Finally, below the doomed couple at the bottom of the painting, she'd attached a small bar of motel soap. Carved on the surface, in her distinctive script, was the word SAFE.

I hated leaving Sas's art behind, but my tiny car could not carry everything—my kitchen utensils with which I'd learned how to cook, paintings and sculpture from all my artist pals; my library, my flower garden; my students at the college, my scientists at Los Alamos, the elders at Pueblo; the warmth of the Spanish language, the smell of burning piñon, my rivers, my trout, my sunsets over the mesa, the Sangre de Cristo Mountains, my snowstorms and thunderstorms, and a stream of friends who didn't even know I was leaving.

I slept fitfully, holding Badger and Callie close, my ear cocked for the Trooper coming up the driveway or noises on my patio. I awoke at dawn and peeked out the window. Trey's car was nowhere to be seen.

I threw in what I'd packed the night before, hastily stuffed both cats into the back seat, and shut the car door. I checked my house one last time. Before locking up I hesitated, then quickly lifted Sas's piece from the wall.

When I opened the car to get in, Callie shot out and raced toward the juniper bushes.

I chased after her, not going to the place in my brain that said I might have to leave her behind. But the sun was coming up and I did not want to encounter Trey arriving or any scene that might follow.

"Callie," I whispered, my heart aching and at the same time visualizing dropping her into a cat stew.

"Callieeeeeee…" She disappeared into the huge juniper grove on the west side of the house. I scrambled underneath the prickly branches on my hands and knees. I crept closer, but she scampered deeper into the underbrush. A car on the nearby road slowed down, and I heard gravel crunching beneath its wheels. I willed Callie toward me and, inching toward her, finally managed to lure her into my hands and backed out of the underbrush while pieces of dead juniper fell down into my shirt and bra. I dived toward my car, looking neither right nor left. Badger's mustached face peered out of the driver's window. I threw Callie in, slammed the door, and turned on the ignition. She yowled, and Badger hissed at her. Any final view I might have had of the Rocking H was clouded by tears.

Heading out of town and across the mesa, my once-enchanted life grew smaller and smaller in my rearview mirror. When I reached the Gorge Bridge, I slowed down and craned to look over the edge of the guardrail. Far below, the river roared as it always had, and I imagined the trout in their pools poised for their morning caddis hatch. I hit the gas, and when I reached the other side, the vast expanse of desert stretched before me, as did the sixteen-hundred-mile journey back to the Pacific Northwest, the home I'd left so long ago.

I glanced over at Sas's collage on the passenger seat, its coral hues even more radiant outside of my dark bedroom. The inscription on the soap spoke to me like a talisman, but the truth was I had no idea what lay ahead. My terra firma had cracked wide open, and now I was that falling stone in the Gorge. Though I knew where I was going to land, I didn't know how hard.

PART II:
LAND OF FORGETTING

Chapter 15.

⟨Glory Be to God for Dappled Things⟩

I'D LONGED FOR A HORSE as far back I could remember. The year I turned twelve, Mom and Dad finally caved in. Since I was what they called a "willful child," I imagine they relented partially because of their concerns where that "will" might take me, but my mother had grown up with horses, and she was quietly excited. On Mom's dressing table was a framed black-and-white photo of her as a smiling teenager standing next to Gay, her beloved bay mare. One time when I was gazing yet again at the photo, she said, "That picture is the real me."

So on a sunny September Saturday Mom, Dad, and I set off to see a chestnut mare for sale. When I sat in the saddle she stood patiently and responded softly to the bit. By the time I'd ridden her down the driveway, I was certain she was the horse for me: pretty, easy to ride, and, according to Mom, "not too expensive."

"Plus, we could breed her," Mom said, smiling back at me from the front seat. I couldn't believe my ears. Everything I'd dreamed of and more. A colt, too!? I was sold.

By the time we got home, it was settled. We told Paul and Rosemary about the mare, and when Dad called the owners, we were all excited, even Paul who wasn't the least bit interested in horses. He rallied, though, imagining a horse looking in our back door like Mr. Ed.

When Dad returned from the phone, his face said it all.

"I'm sorry," he said, not looking at me. "The mare is sold. Right after we left, someone came and wrote a check."

I could barely move. Tears burned my eyes. How could this be possible? Especially when it all seemed so perfect?

"Well," Mom said quietly, closing the novel on her lap, "I guess there's something better waiting for you, then...."

By October, after many unsuitable candidates, my mother had enlisted my grandfather, Boppa, in the horse search. He'd steered clear of our quest, which puzzled Mom, but now I can see why: he knew how much was wrapped up in having horses; it wasn't like getting a cat from the shelter. But my mother finally convinced Boppa to help, and by the following weekend he, Mom, Dad, and I were on our way to a small town in the foothills of the Cascade Mountains where the Stillaguamish River blasts out of glacial runoff. We were meeting Frank Melang, an old horse friend of Boppa's. Apparently, Frank had an Arabian gelding for sale. When we pulled up at his driveway, he was waiting in an old red pickup. We all shook hands as Boppa introduced us, and then Frank turned to me. "The horse is in a herd several miles up the valley in another field. Why don't you ride with me?" I looked at Mom and Dad and they nodded. "We'll follow you," Dad said and smiled.

I jumped into the cab of Frank's truck, which smelled of cigarettes, leather, and hay. We bumped down the washboard road, then rounded a long curve that hugged the raging river. The road opened up into a huge meadow where vine maple blazed red-orange along the cliffs above. After another mile along the edge of the field, we all stopped and got out near a gate just as the low-slung autumn sun peeked over the mountains. No sign of horses. Fog hovered over the grass, and our breath came out in big puffs. Frank lifted his fingers to his mouth, letting out a whistle that echoed off the mountains. Silence. Just the whistle bouncing back off the river.

First a rumble. Low at first, then it grew, as if the boulders on Mt. Pilchuck were tumbling down its face. "Oh…," we murmured, until the source of the sound came round the stand of yellow birches. A herd of twenty or thirty horses, many with black spots and splashes of white, galloped toward us at full speed, the ground shaking, their breath like smoke in the cold morning air. Out in front, leading them all, a dappled, dark-gray Arabian, his head held high, red nostrils flaring, his magnificent tail held high.

"That's him," Frank said. I held my breath. I'd never seen such a horse in all my life. When the horses slowed to a trot, they came straight for us, milling and huffing around Frank, who offered them a handful of oats from his pocket. The gray pushed the others away and came right up to Frank's chest. "So. This is Colonel Glenn." Frank patted his neck. "But we call him Lightfoot." He pointed to the hind fetlock, the only flash of white on his otherwise dark legs.

"I'm trying to introduce Arabian blood into my Appaloosa herd," Frank said. "Lightfoot's a good example of what that can do. He didn't get the Appaloosa spots, but he sure got the Arabian confirmation." My mother had told me about how Arabians had dished faces and wide-set eyes and high-held tails. Frank smoothed Lightfoot's mane and Lightfoot nodded, nosing Frank's pocket.

"I named him after the astronaut John Glenn." Frank laughed. "The night Glenn blasted off into space for the first time, my wife shouted out to the barn to come in and watch on television. 'I can't!' I yelled, 'I'm delivering a foal!'" We all laughed. It did not surprise me that this horse was connected to the stars.

When Frank saddled Lightfoot, he gave me a leg up, and all the power of that herd seemed harnessed into one horse. Coiled and electric like hope, danger, and possibility rolled into one. His delicate ears pointed ahead, and when I touched his belly with my heel, his gait was quick and snappy like my brother's caps on the Fourth of July. This was no chestnut mare or, as Mom would later say, "not just another brown horse."

"He's only green broke, even though he's six," Frank said. "Not much training. He doesn't know about cars or anything like that. But he doesn't have a mean bone in his body." He rubbed Lightfoot's handsome face.

Dad asked Frank a few questions. He'd had no experience with horses except with Mom on her farm during their college summers, but he wondered if Lightfoot was going to be too much horse for me. Frank agreed that Lightfoot was not a quiet, cold-blooded horse, but Mom and I exchanged an eyebrows-up, conspiratorial *yes*. Boppa just stood back and puffed his pipe, a quiet smile on his lips. I knew what he was thinking: *This was a fine horse.* When Mom quoted Gerard Manley Hopkins, "Glory be to God for dappled things," I leaned forward in the saddle and touched Lightfoot's shoulder, knowing I could not imagine another horse in all the solar system. On that cold October morning, desert blood filled my veins.

A hot-blooded horse and a wet Pacific Northwest forest, however, are not always the best combo. Lightfoot adjusted well to the move from the mountains to the sea, but the trails were overgrown, and I often wore a big rubber poncho to keep the rain off us both. Plus, Lightfoot's high spirits had been a big challenge for me. That first winter, he'd spooked from a backfiring truck and run away with me down a snowy hill, my long, blonde pigtails flying behind me. My love for him had nothing to do with girly notions of ribbons in manes or plastic horse statues on knickknack shelves. (Those were the same girls who dreamed about being a princess.) For me a horse was about being one with a creature who could carry me across the wide, wide earth. It went with my need to carry a pocketknife in my jeans at all times, and to wear my studded cowboy belt. I'd managed to prove to my parents I could handle this gallant creature.

The Arabian horse is the oldest existing breed in the world. In fact, every horse on the planet has a bit of Arabian DNA. Like humans, these horses originated in the desert, and their interaction with people can be traced back over four thousand years. Their black skin (no matter which coat color) protected them from the harsh sun. Bred for speed and stamina, they developed a huge lung capacity, too. They also possess one fewer vertebra than other breeds—which gives them shorter, stronger backs. Unusually intelligent, thoughtful, and hot-blooded, they were valued for their ability to think as well as survive in harsh circumstances. The Bedouins needed their horses to be alert and strategic when carrying warriors into battle, often traveling hundreds of miles across the desert sands. I learned all this, of course, from Boppa's books like *Drinkers of the Wind*, one of my favorites and my mother's, too. Even though Lightfoot wasn't a purebred, he had a pedigree I traced back several generations. I got my hands on an Arabic language dictionary and translated his name to "Moud'i Q'adam," "light-of-foot": ال قدم مو ضي. The swirls in the characters echoed the shapes of my horse's mane.

What I loved most about the history of the Arabian, though, along with what sounded like an exotic life in the desert, was how the Bedouins treated their horses. They raised the foals in the tents, feeding them camel's milk and dates. (Just the *sound* of camel's milk and dates is enough to make a teenage girl swoon.) For thousands of years they were members of their human families, dependent on one another to survive the punishing desert. It's speculated that this is why the Arabian horse is so loyal, so sensitive to human emotion.

I counted myself lucky that Dad had remodeled the garden house as a stable so that Lightfoot could be close to our family. We could all see his head poking out of the stable Dutch door from our kitchen window, just as Paul had predicted. After school I'd bring my horse home from my friend's big field down the road where he grazed during the day, then go for a long ride. Lightfoot's presence at home added to Mom's dream, too, I think. Our Meadowdale house near the beach was built by an Englishman as a nursery. The three acres included a 1920s gray clapboard house, the small gardener's house (Lightfoot's stable), and burgeoning exotic plants and trees landscaped into secret gardens. Banks of rhododendrons lined the curvy driveway that cut through Japanese maples and sweet gum trees. There was even a pond with an old arched, stone bridge. A fountain in the middle froze in winter and created an ice sculpture that we petted as we skated on our boots across the frozen pond.

Meadowdale was actually a kind of miniature Manderley, a Daphne du Maurier dream for my mother. She reveled in her vegetable garden, her flowers, and the old patio where we grilled salmon in the summer. She'd tip her head and say, "Listen," as her favorite summer bird, the Swainson's thrush, sang his wavery tremolo. Occasionally Dad lured her away on one of his business trips to San Francisco or Hawaii, but Mom always preferred being home with her animals and children. "It might be hard for my roses…," she'd say. "And besides, my house will miss me if I'm gone."

The woods behind our house stretched up a hill, and they contained lots of mysterious trails as well as pheasants who chimed their echoey calls. The occasional skunk would appear, too. And we never saw him, but once a porcupine shot several quills into our dog Captain's nose. After riding Lightfoot on the beach and up the dirt roads where we could canter, I wanted my new horse to see the secret place I loved, a clearing at the top of our woods we called "The Lookout," where my father had lashed railroad ties over an old rotten well. We'd always been warned not to mess with the sturdy cover he'd built.

Lightfoot and I slithered over the mossy bridge. The cedars hung low over the rotten logs, the spongy trail disappeared under overhanging blackberry bushes, and Lightfoot snorted at the devil's club and rustling alder trees. I was living my dream, though, crossing the West (albeit a moist and green one) on my trusty horse. Just as he followed me everywhere in the pasture, Lightfoot willingly forged ahead where I asked him, and, in the six months he'd been mine, we'd already covered miles of Puget Sound trails, roads, and beaches.

About twenty feet after the bridge, the path unexpectedly turned into a slick, oozy swamp. Lightfoot's legs began to thrash. I held onto his mane as he struggled to stay upright. He thrashed again, and the mud sucked us down. Skunk cabbage, flagrant in its primordial bloom, stank like fear itself. I'd had enough spooky moments with Lightfoot to know that a frightened horse cannot think straight. Just the sheer size of a calm horse is enough to worry some people, but now I had one thousand pounds of horse fighting a deepening mire. Lightfoot's hoofprints were filling rapidly with the oily-blue water from the swamp. How could I have known that my safe and familiar forest could contain such a trap?

I loosened the reins, thinking he might instinctively get himself out, but he groaned, and the sucking sounds grew louder as he tried in vain to escape the slime. "Oh please, God…," I cried out loud. "Please help us." Suddenly I spied a huckleberry bush growing out of a rotten stump near dry ground. I swung off Lightfoot and leapt to grab a branch. I landed near the base of the stump and scrabbled up the roots, still managing to clutch one rein.

"Come on, boy. Come on, fella," I tried to coax him toward me, my voice trembling like Lightfoot's body. Adrenaline pumped through my veins, and the whites of Lightfoot's eyes were wild. Then in an act of my own instinct, I dropped the reins and scampered around the perimeter of the swamp till I was behind my horse. In the midst of panic, I was able to holler with deep and utter force, "Get up! Get on, boy!! Get on!!" stamping my foot and waving my arms to startle him forward.

That did it. In one surge—and no small amount of his own adrenaline—Lightfoot lurched and staggered out, his legs slick and black, mud spattered on me, on his belly, the cinch, even the nearby salmonberries. We both stood there quivering, I with a sense of relief. But then I noticed his back-left leg, the one he was named for, the sole white sock on an otherwise dark dappled-gray body. Except it wasn't white. It was black, mixed with dark red. He held up his leg and shook it as the blood dripped onto the pine needles on the forest floor.

"Oh, oh, oh, no," my heart contracted with fear and remorse for what I'd asked of my horse. "Oh, Lightfoot…" I reached down to touch his fetlock. Straight out from the pastern joint, right above the hoof, protruded a stick the size of a half-smoked cigarette. In all the commotion, he must have jammed his joint against a submerged log. Blood continued to flow.

Holding my breath, I led him step by limping step away from the Lookout Trail, back over the bridge, down the upper pasture, past the vegetable garden to the backyard where I shouted, "Mom! Mom! Come quick!" My mother raced out the back door, dish towel in hand. She took one look at Lightfoot's condition and we exchanged silent glances. "Don't look, honey," she said, patting Lightfoot gently on his flank, then leaned down and using the dish towel to get purchase, in one swift yank, she pulled the stick out of Lightfoot's no-longer-light foot. Lightfoot flinched and whinnied softly, nodding his head.

"Get me some hydrogen peroxide," Mom said. We washed the bloody wound, unsaddled and brushed him, then put him in the stable. That night Lightfoot's foot swelled to the size of a cantaloupe.

Mom said the stick had obviously penetrated a delicate joint. I knew right then I wouldn't be riding him for a long, long time.

The vet arrived with a twitch in his hand, its chain at the end of the stick. "Oh, no," I said. "He doesn't need that."

"This will keep him calm," the vet said, shaking as he administered the tool that looked more like a medieval instrument of torture. A twitch around a horse's upper lip can touch a pressure point and release endorphins to calm him in a medical procedure, but I could see Lightfoot was afraid of the vet himself. He was forcing the twitch, using it as a punishment, forcing my horse to stamp and roll his eyes. Lightfoot was not difficult; in fact, he'd been very patient with everything since the accident. The vet took a look at the foot and prescribed liniment that I was to administer morning and night, presumably to take down the swelling.

So every day before school and all afternoon, I sat in the sawdust of Lightfoot's stall, rubbing and massaging the pepperminty solution into my horse's swollen leg. He shook a bit but often turned his head around to nose me while I wept and rubbed, wept and rubbed, trying to harbor some grim hope that I would ride my precious desert horse again.

Chapter 16.

❦ Connecting Cord ❦

"ZIMBABWE IS ON THE RIGHT-HAND side of the Kalahari Desert." My mother's notes to herself were scattered everywhere—on the coffee table, stuffed in her pockets and dresser drawers. Even in the laundry room. "*Son, Paul. Senior Editor, Harvard Business Review, Boston, Mass.*" Then in pencil after this (circled): "*11:32 PM to bed.*" One note surfaced with the word "*BARN,*" followed by "*ON WAY HOME WHITE OWL ON WIRE.*" I was baffled until I recalled that I'd told her how, driving home from New Mexico, my headlights had illuminated a barn owl who swooped so close to my car I could have touched him. Since I'd arrived home, Mom's memory loss seemed to accelerate. Though she was a note-taker her whole life, the random scribblings around the house became more and more disjointed, especially disturbing since language was my mother's compass.

"I love novels," she'd always say, peeking over the top of *Far from the Madding Crowd* or *Pride and Prejudice*. "They take you right inside how other people think." When Paul, Rosemary, and I were in school she'd welcomed detailed accounts of our days ("Okay, *First* Period…"), offering a thoughtful response to whatever victory or crisis loomed at the moment. We'd sit on the big couch in our living room in Meadowdale, legs curled beneath us, or at the kitchen table, and go over the minutiae again and again: Should I enter Lightfoot in the winter 4-H Furry Coat Horse Show? How could Rosemary avoid getting stomachaches when her second grade teacher Mrs. Laycock brought grisly news stories to share with the class? Was J. D. Salinger's Holden Caulfield really a version of the author? Even in adult life, everything from boyfriend problems to my brother's law school applications were dissected, examined, and commented upon, by all five of us. My mother would quote Yeats when she got up from reading to make a meal: "I will arise and go now, and go to Innisfree," she'd say, making her way to the stove.

Both my parents believed in the power of words. "Write it down!" my father would say if we were troubled by something. "Write it down, then write a solution." He often taped tidy pieces of notepaper to the bathroom mirror where he shaved. Things like *"FOUR POUNDS OVER: LOSE FOUR POUNDS"* (all caps, just as he typed) and listed below were dates and measurements of his progress.

As a child I couldn't imagine writing down *"lost Alfie"* since I already knew my stuffed turtle was missing, and I didn't have a solution, but my father was all about solving things by getting them out in the open; if it was on paper, it was not glooming around in our heads. He also had a broad-brushstroke solution for worry in general. If, for example, my brother was yet again behind in one of his articles for the high school paper and bemoaning the possibility of getting fired, my father would boom, "What will *happen?*" swiping away every possible disastrous outcome with a simple existential question. Then he'd press the point. "What is the *worst* possible thing if you get fired? Will you *die?*" The final possibility seemed rather extreme in proportion to my brother's late article, but he'd continue, "And if *that* happened," he paused for emphasis, "is that such a bad thing? Really?" My father's assurance that even death itself wasn't the end-all revealed the breadth of his confidence.

Whether his idea of death was heaven or just the next adventure, he was emboldened by erasing it from his list of problems. And even if it was just his attempt to control life's chaos, his positive mindset was a law of nature in the Hemp family.

When I limped home from Riojos that fall, I truly believed I was coming back to the land of "What Will Happen?!" and all its attendant problem-solving relief. Needless to say, I was disoriented by the ripped-Band-Aid departure from New Mexico, so finding my mother—the mistress of detail—asking the same questions over and over felt like a reprise of the altered reality I'd left behind. "So where did you say Trey was? Why hasn't he called? What happened in Riojos? Why did you come home?"

There are times in life when, after a sustained period of uncertainty, the right action becomes clear. Whether it's a survival response or an inner voice you cannot ignore, you act. At that time, you're convinced that this event—the one that made you act—is the whole story and it will define you forever. Down the road, however, you discover that "it" isn't the real story at all, merely the bellwether of a larger narrative. It seems preposterous to compare one's own tiny life with human history, but if we back up, the arc of each life appears as a miniature of the human story: random events, struggles of power, plagues, healing, violence, war, and rejuvenation. Death.

One of the most profound things I learned in college still sticks with me: History is not merely a series of happenings, and those happenings are not necessarily the "cause" of events that follow. Those occurrences rise out of what philosopher T. S. Kuhn called a "climate of opinion," the paradigm of the times. Think the Austro-Hungarian Archduke Ferdinand's assassination; Pearl Harbor; Princess Diana's tragic death in a car wreck; jets plowing into the World Trade Center; a suspect presidential election that shocks and bitterly divides a country. In and of themselves, these events look like the *reasons* for what comes after. We hover over them, reliving every detail, clutching and dissecting, as if by doing so we will understand. According to Kuhn, though, they're indicators of something much larger going on underneath. Canaries in the mine.

For me, I couldn't see it then (I was still flailing around for words to explain it to myself), but Trey's final meltdown and my hasty exit turned out to be the booster rocket that shot me out of his gravitational pull. For a long time, of course, I considered that drama the biggest disaster of my life (aren't we always the center of our own story?!) and continued to cast Trey as a predator, the thief of my beloved town and friends. And in some ways he was, but later I came to see my departure from Riojos as a backhanded blessing, a gift from Trey. It prepared me for things to come.

In the months after leaving New Mexico, I never once heard from the falconer. No phone call. No letter. Not a whisper of an email. Nothing. The only hint of his existence was my monthly bank statement, which had been forwarded a month after I'd left. I noticed that our joint checking account had been closed, the remaining $25.38 withdrawn, a fact I observed more in sorrow than in anger.

At first, I'd stayed at Rosemary's house near Seattle, cuddling baby Celia and accepting her husband Freddie's vodka tonics. My sister fixed up the guest bedroom with a desk and cozy comforters. But Badger and Callie needed to have a more permanent space, so eventually I camped out at my parents' new condo across Puget Sound. I spent hours on the phone weeping to my friends about the injustice of it all, shuttling between outrage and self-pity. Friends in Riojos reported they had run into Trey, his hair a mess and a crazed look in his eye. One friend had spotted him at an art opening, and she, not knowing I'd left town, asked how I was. He'd told her I was back at the Rocking H Ranch working on deadline for a magazine article. An even more alarming story came from a friend who'd attended a local reading where he recited lovesick poems he'd written about me and his empty bed. Someone else said Trey had taken up writing art criticism. Finally, I told my friends: no more news about Trey. Period. Paragraph.

When my father couldn't take my weeping any longer ("I will help you find a place to live; I'll contribute the first month's rent; I'll help you move! But please—can you just stop crying?"), I landed a shingled, one-room beach cottage perched on the northern edge of the Olympic Peninsula, just an hour north from my parents' place. With Dad's help, I moved a couple of pieces of furniture from family storage and began a new life in a new town.

One evening several months after coming home, I urged my father to spend the weekend away, and I went to stay overnight with Mom. In the last year Dad had closed his consulting business called Travel Marketing, Inc. He still kept his office for his own projects, but he'd been so much looking forward to hiking and traveling with Mom, writing columns for the local paper about the Olympic Peninsula, and doing some long-distance road trips on his own. Clearly that wasn't happening, but at least I could give him a break.

When I arrived at the condo, I found books by Mom's favorite authors—Iris Murdock, Thomas Hardy, Jane Austen, Anne Tyler, and Eudora Welty—stacked near her bed, obviously their physical proximity a source of comfort. After dinner she sat at the dining room table with William Saroyan's *My Name Is Aram* open in front of her, mouthing sentences. I had no idea if she comprehended them; I just let her read. She always valued not only the meaning of words, but their beauty, as if their aesthetic power could protect us from incivility or degradation. Even the shapes of letters themselves offered her a handhold. Now, however, I could see that she was losing her grip on language itself.

The next morning, she held out a yellow-lined piece of paper with bold printing in my father's hand. "What's this?" she said. I looked at the paper: "*TODAY CHRISTINE IS HERE.*" I took it from her and explained that Dad was not being condescending, that he was just helping her with the day's schedule. "Remember how he likes his lists, Mom," I chirped. I could not say, "Mom, are you crazy? Dad showed this to you last night before he left!" So I put my arm around her wondering what exactly was happening to us, our family. I seemed to have traded one loony place for another.

"Okay," she said, "but what does *this* mean? Who wrote THIS?!" She held out another note, written to Dad on the back of blue gift-wrapping paper stamped with Beatrix Potter bunnies. The following words were formed in my mother's distinctive, lacy handwriting:

> Hi Peter - I went into the big bathroom and lo and BE
> HOLD found <u>some kind of animal</u> who <u>disappeared quickly</u> but
> 'he' <u>must still be somewhere</u> near that door.
> BE Care—Full
> Love,
> You

Though I knew no one in my new little seaside town, the landscape was utterly familiar. Moss and kelp. Overgrown blackberries and sea grasses. Gray skies. Out of the Straits rose Whidbey Island, the back side of which I'd seen from my bedroom window as a child. Other than the dining room table and a childhood dresser Dad and I had moved, my new digs were pretty spare, but Rosemary came to the rescue. She drove the two-hour trip, including ferry crossing, from Seattle to bring plates and tea kettles, pans and a bread maker. One day she arrived, and I was still in my pajamas, wool socks, and the puce-colored wool hat I'd bought because I couldn't seem to sleep without layers of padding. Rosemary drew the line at the hat. "Not your best look," she said, lugging a microwave into the kitchen.

Celia's blonde hair smelled like baby soap, and I snuggled her on a pile of blankets by the woodstove while my sister prepared a bottle. Chamber music came in loud and clear on Canadian radio. The winter wind whipped down the eaves, and whitecaps charged across the Straits. Rosemary bundled up Celia for a walk as I told her about being alone in this wild place, sleeping in the tiny loft on a futon. I'd tacked some carpet samples to the ladder so Badger and Callie could climb up and sleep with me. Then I burst into tears.

"Get dressed now," Rosemary told me, slipping Celia into her tiny, blue rubber boots. "And truly, Sister, there will be a time when you have created a life beyond Riojos, beyond the hawk." She'd heard me tell her over and over that my life had come to a dead end, that I could think of nothing except my anger and my sorrow and what-could-have-been. She looked up from zipping Celia's rain jacket. "It's actually better that it happened in one clean departure." She snugged mittens on Celia's hands. "At least it was clear what you had to *do.*" We put Celia into the stroller and headed out into the wind and rain.

"But I'm still wondering if I could have done something *more,* something *else* to make it *right*…," I said, hurrying to keep up with my sister, who always walks with great purpose. Rosemary is tall, like me but with short black hair, which was turning early gray. She moves in quick, direct spurts. As a child she walked tilting forward, as if her legs could not keep up with her brain. She was always thinking ahead. Right after I arrived tattered from Riojos, she'd trotted me straight to a loss-support group. ("You have to grieve properly," she'd said. "Trey. The babies. Your old life. Everything.")

Celia chattered in the stroller, and seagulls coasted in the air along the beach. "Well," Rosemary muscled the stroller over a grassy hump, "your friends in Riojos are saying that Trey's telling everyone he's 'lost the love of his life,' but he hasn't even called! You'd think he'd want to know where you are, at least!" We followed the trail up into the woods where huge maple leaves collaged yellow-brown patterns on the path. "I mean—it isn't as if he left his scarf at a concert."

I didn't tell her how often he appeared in my dreamlife, and that I couldn't seem to scare him out. Even his ghoulish dead father made appearances.

"Can you at least tell me again, though?" I asked my sister, "that I've done the *right thing*?" Pathetic as it was, I needed to hear it once more.

"Of course you did," Rosemary said. Her voice, brisk and sure, reminded me of my mother and how she'd find, even in the dullest days, something to look forward to. Driving in the dreary rain after a childhood dentist appointment, she might say, "Oh, let's just go home, cozy in, and have a nice sandwich, shall we?" Or, on a family vacation, if there was not a good picnic spot for a lunch stop, she'd say, "Let just park by this nice bush."

When Rosemary, Celia, and I emerged from the forest, a small flock of geese, stragglers in the southbound migration, flew above us. I swallowed my tears. My sister, like the lifetime partnered goose, seemed so at home in her marriage, in her little family. How had she done it? I'd always harbored a mild aversion to her suburban lifestyle: mortgage, jazzercise classes, trips to Target. Freddie, a plumbing contractor, loved providing the comforts of such a life, especially after Rosemary took time off as a television writer and producer in order to raise her baby. She went to a parent-baby group, dropped off baskets of fruit for friends whose children were sick. She did volunteer jobs at the homeless shelter for her church.

I'd lived so long in the rarefied air of small communities from Vermont to London, from Boston to Riojos, where aesthetics and lean living were valued above dishwashers and garbage disposals. A cul-de-sac life had always terrified me.

Rosemary turned the stroller around, so the wind would be at our backs. "Right now you feel like everything revolves around your pain. But what did that friend in Riojos say? 'Time is a gentleman.'" Celia kicked her feet out of the blanket, her peachy face like a putto in a Renaissance altarpiece. I tucked her tighter into the buggy.

"And wouldn't you rather be with someone you can live *with* instead of someone you *can't live without*?" Rosemary turned up the hill toward my cottage. "It's like a painting. Years from now, this part of the picture will only be one little corner, a fern in the forest." When we got to the porch I hoisted Celia from the stroller, she clinging to my neck, her breath sweet and warm. She had inherited my blonde hair and my proclivity for talk. Her prelanguage phrases skipped up and down the scale, imitating Rosemary's and my conversation not in words, but in consonants and vowels, a sing-songy story made clear by the cadences and pauses alone—what Robert Frost might have called "the sound of sense." As we opened the door, met by Badger and Callie, Rosemary said, "Why don't we all just cozy in and have some nice soup?"

Rosemary's presence in my tiny cottage reminded me that love, like making art, is a sacred vocation. They're both enacted in times of passion and elation, yes, but much of the work must be done when one is least inspired. I guessed that's why Christian monks and nuns have their daily offices, rabbis a disciplined study of the Torah; Muslims kneel daily toward Mecca, and Buddhists sit in meditation. All practices are quiet preparation for the (rare) moments of glory. Like an ascetic in the desert, the artist must stay focused lest she be tempted by the demons of procrastination (otherwise known in my family as "the lure of the horizontal").

Not long after Rosemary and Celia went home, a cold wind charged down the Straits from Alaska. I fed the stove, slapped yet another Portuguese Fado CD in my stereo, and basked in my sorrows. Until the phone rang.

"I called your number in Riojos, but a recording gave me this one." It was Gary, an old friend from Boston. "Where *are* you exactly? What's going on?" His voice was urgent. "The launch is next month! Where's that poem?!"

In the mad dash of leaving Riojos, I'd actually forgotten about Gary's project. Ten years earlier, he and I were out to dinner when he'd casually mentioned he'd received a grant from NASA.

"NASA? Great!" I said, still glowing from a thousand-dollar Massachusetts Arts Grant I'd received that year. "How much?"

"Uh, 33 million dollars." He reached for the salt.

Gary was an astrophysicist and had designed a miniature observatory to record the prenatal activity of stars. It was called SWAS, short for Submillimeter Wave Astronomy Satellite, and was meant to reveal what happens before they begin to twinkle, a kind of stellar ultrasound.

"I think a poem of yours should be part of this mission," Gary wiped his mouth with his napkin.

"Wow," I said, looking up from my spaghetti. "Apparently you don't have to *be* a rocket scientist to send a poem into space; you just have to *know* one."

"That's right," Gary folded his napkin. "So get busy."

For Gary, getting a rocket off the ground, however, was like trying to get a book of poems published. The project faced many false starts. After the satellite was completed, scheduling problems at NASA delayed the launch for four more years—which is why I'd forgotten about it. That night, when I told Gary about Trey and my escape from New Mexico, all he could say was, "Houston, we have a problem."

I pulled on my puce hat, and for the next few days I went to work. I scrapped the stiff, ponderous poem I'd composed years before, and when the new poem emerged, it was about stars, yes, but it turned out to be about something else. I called the poem "Connecting Cord."

> When a child is waiting
> to be born, light shines
> inside. No one
> but the mother knows
> what trembles there…She's the blanket, the safe
> cloud, hiding her pin-point
> of glittery possibility…

Before I FedExed it to Gary, though, I called him to ask what kind of paper to print it on.

"Just spray it with Raid," he said. "You never know who might be reading it out there in space…And," (as if I had no choice) "you need to come see the launch."

Vandenberg Air Force Base stretches out on the rocky California coast, about three hours north of Los Angeles. Huge frames of space shuttle gantries stood like sentinels on the nearby hill, but SWAS, buried inside a smaller Pegasus rocket, was to be launched from the underbelly of a Lockheed 1011 jet. It seemed fitting that my poem would be carried into space by a horse with wings.

With my NASA clearance card at the ready and wearing a static-grounding strap on my boot (too much compressed fuel to joke about sparks), I made my way to the "hot pad." I patted the rocket. Apparently, my poem had been transferred to foil to protect it from the heat of the blastoff, then stowed deep inside the womb of the satellite's observatory. For the first time in several months, my attention was on something other than my own sorry heart. At sunset Gary and I held our breath as the jet lifted the rocket—tucked safely under the fuselage—into the sky. After ten years of work, these scientists were ready to see their baby born. For Gary, the launch embodied much of his adult life's work. Though I was not exactly crucial to the project, I, too, was invested in a larger trajectory: I was birthing my poem into the cosmos.

After the plane was airborne, Gary and I raced back into the control center to sit on console with the team to watch our precious cargo from a remote camera secured to the plane. The countdown ticked, the anticipation palpable. Then, at five minutes before the drop, a scratchy voice came through our headphones, "ABORT! ABORT!" Gary's face was stricken.

The voice burst through, "RECYCLE. RECYCLE," apparently the command to return to base. For an absurd moment I imagined something wrong with the poem and NASA officials saying, "This line doesn't scan...." But the glitch turned out to be a software problem, and the satellite was forced to come down.

Gary didn't know whether the next launch would be the next day or the next week. Deflated, I sat in my hotel room and watched *Mister Rogers' Neighborhood* on PBS, his kind voice like a salve. Gary called and said gloomily there was still no news about the launch schedule; it could be weeks before it would fly again.

Since I was maxed out on my credit card, I packed up and drove back to Los Angeles, indulging in yet another jag of tears. When I pulled into the constellation of cars at the LAX rental lot, I was startled into my senses: If I were to fly back to Seattle now, then what had I come here for? Was I going to abandon my poem right as it teetered on the brink of being star-born? That little piece of me stowed in a Pegasus rocket was a living being itself. I needed to "recycle," go back—no matter what the cost—to see my poem thunder into space. What was money compared to that? I could hear my father's can-do voice booming, "Why not!?"

Without consulting the attendant, I turned the car around, negotiated my way out of the tangle of satellite roads, pointed my car north, and drove the four hours back to Vandenberg. I checked back into the hotel and called Gary.

"It flies tomorrow," he said.

The launch day dawned cold and clear. Out my hotel room window, the pale-blue sky hovered over the coast like a movie set. I dressed quickly and met my now-familiar comrades who were preparing for a sunset launch. All day we watched the sky, hoping for no clouds, no wind. The weather held. When evening came, once again the Lockheed 1011 rolled down the runway, and we held our breath as it lifted for the sky. This time we drove nervously back to the control tower, not allowing ourselves the luxury of excitement.

My heart began to beat faster at five minutes and counting. Soon we heard, "10, 9, 8, 7, 6, 5, 4, 3, 2, 1…"

When the voice in the headset said, "DROP," white light filled the monitor screens, and a deafening shout rose in the control room. I ripped off my headphones and raced downstairs and outside. Sure enough, swimming across the shimmery sky, the rocket carrying the satellite glinted in the setting sun, its winged contrail sweeping behind it, booster rockets exploding, the sunset turning it pink. We whooped and waved our arms, following the vessel with our eyes—up up up. And then it was gone, heading straight for the stars. All that remained was a squiggly white line in its wake, its own poem in the sky.

When I returned home, I immediately called Mom to report my poem's epic journey. "Oh! That sounds wonderful!" she said. "And what poem are you talking about?"

Chapter 17.

⌒ *Coming Home* ⌒

"It's really all about memory," Ken says. He jumps up on the fence, balances on the top rail, and adjusts his water-stained canvas hat. "It's the past that makes Buddy think he needs to escape instead of listening to you."

We are working on very subtle cues for Buddy to modulate his gait, but Buddy just wants to rush, as if going faster would relieve his stress. I tell Ken about Buddy's wild trot when I am riding.

"When he's nervous he goes right into that default," Ken says. I stand in the middle of the ring and cluck to Buddy. His ear has yet to turn toward me as he trots around counterclockwise.

"I know you used to think Buddy liked to move fast on the trail. But now we're seeing that he'd really rather be relaxed."

"Wouldn't we all?" I say, while continuing to keep my eyes on Buddy as he circles and circles around me in the pen, ignoring any invitation to slow down.

Ken smiles. "Someone once rode the heck out of him. He was running to get away. From the saddle. From the rider. From discomfort. You can show him that he no longer has to do that." I think about how running away had once served me, too.

Buddy trots around tensely, still no ear cocked toward me. Ken says, "Don't pity him, though. He has to find his own way. When he finds it—the calm—when you're both in the music—he will love it. You will love it! Watch for where he finds his body…There! There it is." Buddy shifts into a lovely swinging trot, all four legs moving in unity. His left ear swivels into me as if he's accessed a part of himself that doesn't need to pin his ears back or flee.

"See?" Ken says. Buddy moves freely, relaxed, and continues listening to me with his ear. "And pretty soon he won't be grumpy about this, either. He'll love his job. It will *feel* good to him. He's such a cool horse. He's so smart." I swell with pride and sneak a peek at Ken to see his face while he praises Buddy. But Ken doesn't buy into that.

"Don't get caught up in the emotion of it, Christine, whether it's love or anger or impatience. It gets in the way, and it's not good for Buddy. He's got the stuff to step up to all this, you know. Just be clear. That's all you need to do here. Be clear and consistent. You and Buddy will dance this dance together." I can't help but think of my mother, when one of us kids was naughty or taking up too much space with negative energy: "No casting your gloomy spell!"

Ken swings his other leg over the top rung of the fence and sits on the top rail. "You have a tendency to push him a little bit when you think he's not going to follow though. But don't you dare do the work for him. Don't own his stuff. Stay in the middle and find your own power. It's your responsibility to help him choose the easiest, calmest way. Then ask him to come home."

Ken's words triggered unexpected tears, and I turn my face so he can't see. What is it about Buddy, about opening myself to this horse stuff that leaves me open to such a river of feeling? Ken tells me not to get caught up in the emotion of it, but I can't help myself. All those feelings I've stowed away for decades surge through me like a fast current on the river.

Chapter 18.

The Red Pony

LIGHTFOOT'S INJURY BROUGHT INTO BOLD relief how quickly life can take a horrible turn. I shouldered guilt about my role in the accident. Shouldn't I have scouted out the trail first on foot? I'd always protected my animals, safely shutting my hens in at night, keeping my parakeet Max away from drafts, and calling our Samoyed Captain away from the cars when he followed us to the beach. I'd had goats and rabbits, fish and grasshoppers, cats and chickens, and many had met untimely deaths, accompanied by deep grief, but Lightfoot's injury shook me to the core. I came down with migraines and had to come home from school more than once. Mom didn't mention it, nor did I, but we both knew that lame horses often had to be put down. After a second vet told us the wound must be lanced, Mom said no thank you and went into her own version of problem solving. Unlike my father, who marched boldly toward answers by sheer force, Mom was a ruminator, a researcher. She read. She got on the phone. She asked questions. She sought recommendations. Soon she'd tracked down the best large animal vet in greater Seattle. "Top drawer," she said, after hanging up the phone. "He'll be here on Monday."

The news cheered me, but it scared me, too. What if the fancy vet said there was no hope? What if Lightfoot went the way of John

Steinbeck's red pony? That story was lodged firmly in my family's lore. I'd finished my homework in fifth period study hall one afternoon and had cracked open *The Red Pony*. I was barely into Chapter One when Jan Storvard, a ninth grader, leaned over the table and peered at my book. She was on her way to the bathroom and clutched the hall pass with authority. I quickly covered the open pages with my hands and looked up. From that angle Jan looked unusually large, her white middy blouse accentuating her huge upper arms. Part of me felt sorry for her in her clumpy saddle shoes and ill-fitting pleated skirt. Mom always told us to "be nice to the sad kids"; my siblings and I bore that burden for years. (Why didn't we ever wonder if *we* might be the sad kids?) But Jan was far from pathetic at that moment. "Oh," she whispered, "*The Red Pony*...Hmmmm." She flicked her eyes toward the study hall teacher, then back at me, "Have you come to the part where the pony *dies* yet?" Then she left the room, jiggling the hall pass as the door slammed shut.

It was as if I'd been socked in the belly. Chapter One was now tainted with a terrible foreboding. I sat quietly, my heart beating, while my fellow study-hallers scribbled in their notebooks or gazed out the window at the blooming cherry trees. No matter how hard I tried, I could not erase what I now knew: The Red Pony—to whom I was already deeply attached—was going to die.

When I told my family at the dinner table that night, they all groaned with empathy. Afterward, of course, Jan Storvard's comment became a running theme for spoilers. When Rosemary brought home *James and the Giant Peach* from the school library, Paul said, "Oh—you know the pony dies in the end, don't you?" Or, when I was curled up on the couch with another Will James cowboy novel, Dad, stoking the fire with another chunk of alder, might casually offer, "Doesn't the pony die in that story?"

I hoped the new vet's arrival might also scare away the fears that lurked like the childhood witches in my closet. Strangely, sometimes those fears haunted me even when I was in normal or happy circumstances: in the bathtub or climbing the birch tree that sheltered our whole backyard. Sometimes they'd come in a wave, other times the sensation would sneak up on me in an instant. I'd blink to make sure I was still there, quickly touching our black cat Sandy or the brave kitchen door, my heart racing. I called them my "Not Here Feelings."

My father dealt with such troubles as if they could be managed by an act of will. "Your Not Here Feelings are just an inner ear thing," he'd say, showing me how to put my head down between my knees to get more blood to it. Or, if we were in a blue mood? "Turn the key a quarter turn," he'd say, holding his fingers to his temple, twisting an imaginary key. When I was overwhelmed with long-division problems, due the next morning at school? "Whaddya say we get up at 6:00 a.m., sit at the dining room table, and figure it out? You'll be fresh in the morning." His optimism carried me through the night. Sure enough, at the crack of dawn, we sorted it out, and what had seemed insurmountable the night before was a mere #2 pencil-mark away. For my father, life was a big opportunity, and, as children, we never wanted that to change. In summer, in the long evening light, when the robins cheeped till after ten o'clock, we went to my father to ask for the special favors: "Dad...? Do you think tonight, uh, we could camp out...under the blue spruce by the pond...?" He'd furrow his brow, lean down as if scowling (a good sign), allow for a big, dramatic pause, and then—his visage transformed into possibility—"Whyyyy not?!"

We believed we could always turn something bad into something better, even if it meant occasionally poking fun at a messenger like Jan Storvard. And when situations or stories got too unpleasant or unsavory, my mother would say, "Draw the veil!" and *Old Yeller* (or even an inappropriate joke) would disappear into the ether. In other words, my family did not like sad endings.

When Dr. Nichols stepped out of his shiny white pickup, we knew we were in the presence of a god. He had brown, cropped hair; he wore trim, white coveralls; and the crinkly lines around his eyes gave him a Steve McQueen ruggedness. When he reached out to shake our hands, my mother suddenly got shy. So I told Dr. Nichols the history of the wound. Lightfoot nodded his head while Dr. Nichols stroked his forehead, then casually reached down and handled the fetlock joint with artful grace. Lightfoot reached around and nosed the doc's pocket.

When he'd finished examining the wound, Dr. Nichols shook his head. My heart caved in. Here was the bad news…"That liniment—" he said. "It's exactly the opposite thing to be done with an injury like this." He opened a drawer of his mobile vet unit, pulling out a long needle and syringe. "Cortisone will take down the swelling real soon; it will allow it to heal." He patted Lightfoot gently. No twitch.

"Will he always be lame?" I asked, my voice trembling. Even saying the word was hard for me. The needle moved toward my horse.

Dr. Nichols shook his head and laughed. "Oh, no," he said, patting Lightfoot on the neck. "He might retain some swelling around the fetlock because of that blistering from the liniment, but you'll ride your horse again. Not to worry." He tapped the syringe and gently gave Lightfoot the shot.

Suddenly the spring light seemed to change from sepia to yellow, blue, red, and green. Then Dr. Nichols said, "Now I want you to take him on walks. Every day on a lead. No more standing in the barn all the time. He needs movement to keep his joints and muscles from seizing up. Every day now. Can you do that?" I nodded, grinning madly, unable to hide my glee. Was he kidding!? Of course I could take my horse out of the barn! Of course I could walk him! It's what we loved to do. Bushwhacking. It didn't matter that I wasn't on his back! I could have hugged Dr. Nichols, but I hugged Lightfoot instead. He continued, "You'll have to do this for another month or so, but by summer, he'll be in fine shape." He climbed into his big white truck, started it, and rolled down the window. "I'll be back in two weeks to check on Lightfoot's progress. He'll be sound in no time." Dr. Nichols was right. Not only did Lightfoot heal, he and I went on to win three blue 4-H ribbons at the Snohomish County Fair that year. This time the pony didn't die.

Chapter 19.

∽A Little Bumpy Right Now∽

MY MOTHER'S JAW WAS SET: "Why do I need a person coming into *my* home to look in on me?" Rain poured outside the condo window, obscuring not only Mt. Rainier across the Sound, but the little Kingston harbor below. Mom folded the clean towels on the counter for the fifth or sixth time. Her hands smoothing that cloth were as familiar as her voice and her pretty face framed by her thick, chin-length, silver hair. But today her eyes were worried, and her bangs were pushed aside, revealing a creased brow.

"*My* home?! What does he think he's doing to me?" Mom firmly resisted Dad's efforts to engage an outside person when he went shopping or did errands. It was a big battle between them, yet it was getting riskier to leave her alone, not only for Mom, but for Dad, Rosemary, and me—Celia, too. I was still smarting from a recent night when I'd stayed over with them. After my shower I'd used the lotion in the guest bathroom as a face moisturizer. Within hours my face and neck had broken out in raging hives. The welts swelled around my eyes took a week to subside. Dad and I finally discovered that Mom had filled all the skin lotion bottles with dishwashing detergent.

The kindly wife of one of Dad's friends in the condo complex, Nancy Spicer, had worked with dementia patients. She was a nurse and offered to look in on Mom when Dad was out. Though it was very awkward for him, he'd accepted Nancy's offer a few times. But Mom's home was her temple and her joy. All those years Dad traveled for his business, from Tokyo to Honolulu, Mom had handled everything from tending rose gardens and feeding three children, to wallpapering entire rooms and building kitchen tables. She loved parties and having friends over, but her private time was sacred. When Dad invited Nancy to check on her, the perimeters of her hallowed refuge were transgressed—by her own husband as well as the dreaded Mrs. Spicer.

The big challenge was selling Dad's position without Mom thinking we were taking sides. I couldn't recall having acted as a go-between for my parents before, ever. It was as unfamiliar as Trey's outrageous accusations of betrayal.

"Mom, you've got to give Dad some peace of mind," I told her. "It's for his sake; he worries about you. You know that." Mom fiddled with the dish towel pile.

"It isn't that he's being controlling," I continued, carefully negotiating my way among the thistles. "Though that's what it must feel like. It's a big deal for Dad to ask Nancy to stop in. It's not his style at all." Mom heard the truth in my words and looked up when I said, "He just needs to know you're okay, Mom. Give him that."

She stopped restacking the towels, and her shoulders relaxed as if, to her relief, I'd shown her something new, a break in her resistance. I let it go at that, hoping the conversation would not disappear like the silver napkin rings or the towels she'd flushed down the toilet.

She didn't give in easily, though. At the Ale House that night, she and I had a simple salmon linguine and a glass of white wine. Afterward, Mom nervously looked around the restaurant as if suddenly she were trapped. Her eyes got that worried look again. It was time to take her home. Just as we decided not to order coffee and a sweet, Mom said, "Oh, good. We'll have dessert at home, then." She fussed with the handle of her green purse. "And if there's no ice cream or cookies there…" She paused and looked at me with a twinkle, "We can always drop in at Nancy Spicer's."

The next afternoon I took Mom to the mall. My laptop was having memory problems of its own, something to do with the RAM, and I needed to find a new one. I was determined to make it like our old days of shopping together. We laughed as we got in the car, and I willed the excursion to be smooth, to be good. We jumped around rain puddles in the parking lot and hurried into the surreal world of the superelectronics store. At first Mom was nervous with the noise and commotion. Wall-sized television monitors blared out some daytime talk show and a football game simultaneously. Stereo speakers thumped out a rap tune. Shelf upon shelf of gadgets, cell phones, and printers blinked and shone. The sterile lighting cast no shadows, and pretty soon I found Mom wandering away toward the bright screens, fascinated in a drugged sort of way.

The clerk in the computer aisle fluttered toward us, chirping about the current laptop deals. Mom was clearly getting limp. The woman spoke directly at my mother, oblivious to her condition. "If you need any more help, just look for me or anyone in a blue shirt!" Little did this saleswoman know the magnitude of help we needed. Mom looked down and tugged at the front of her sweater. "I'm wearing a blue shirt."

I veered Mom back toward the laptop aisle, urging her to try the keyboards, and we commented on the different models. Weak with the number of options, I encouraged Mom to consider a silver-blue one I liked, hoping she might have a wise bit of advice. "Nice color," she said, and I flashed to that day years before when she'd come to see me in England. On that road trip we also stopped at Oxford, where I was to study Blake, Keats, and Shelley that summer. We visited the Bodleian Library, where a glass case filled with Shelley relics contained, among other things, a lock of his hair. After taking this in, Mom turned to me and said, "Well, why bother *reading* Shelley…now that we've seen his hair?"

Even as the reality of Mom's dementia settled into our lives, she did seem to retain her sense of irony. One morning I was helping her into her khaki trousers and asked if there was anything else I could get her. She replied, deadpan, "What exactly did you have in mind?" as if I were suggesting a trip to Paris or an intimate dinner party.

Later she and I sat at her dining table having a slice of apple pie. The glass doors were open on a rare early spring day, and the harbor below glittered in the sun. The Olympic Mountains looked so close you could almost reach out your hand and finger the glacier fields. Mom took a bit of pie, then got up yet again to attend to a fly that had been buzzing around us. It got stuck between the window glass and the screen door, its wings flailing. Mom messed with the latch and reached in to rescue it with no success.

"I just don't think he'd be happy in here," she said, after finally shooing the insect out to the fresh air. "Besides, I don't want him eating my pie." She sat down and scooted into the table. "See? I don't have anything to do but flies now."

"It's all relative, Mom," I told her.

"Well," she said, pressing her fork into the pie crust, "You're a relative."

At that moment I realized there must be other powers at work, this ripping me from New Mexico and dropping me back into the heart of my family. At first, I'd thought that my coming home was all about me, but it was becoming clear that more was at stake. Neither my father nor my mother would have demanded I leave my life to help with matters at home, but the timing was uncanny. Mom's crack about the "relative" reminded me of that silly Country Western song "I Come from a Long Line of Love" by Michael

Martin Murphey. Why else would one attend to love's sad and lonely offices? Mom always possessed a philosophical view of misfortune. In the early 1990s she took commuter flights to Walla Walla from Seattle, a pilgrimage she made twice a year to serve on the alumni board of her alma mater, Whitman College. The trip required braving turbulent air over the mountains and down into the thermals of Eastern Washington.

"It's no wonder they call Cascade Airways: 'Crash-cade *Scare*ways,'" Mom reported about a nasty flight across the Cascade Mountains. (Mom hated to fly. Always did.) "From my seat I could see the *pilot* turning green." According to her, the small plane stalled, swayed, and plummeted before regaining equilibrium; then it happened all over again. And again. And again. Meanwhile the jaggy peaks reached up toward the small piece of metal ferrying five people just above the summits.

"How did you make it, Mom?"

"Well…I just *labeled* what was happening at each moment," she explained. "I created a running commentary, so I could distance myself from what seemed like disaster. When the turbulence let up there was a brief, smooth patch. I'd just look out the window and say to myself, 'Oh, it's calm right now…,'" She gave a short laugh. "And when the plane began pitching and diving again, I'd say, 'Hmmmm. It's a little bumpy right now.'" Somehow this helped her get through the last nightmarish half-hour of the trip.

The bumpiness of Mom's dementia, however, was becoming less intermittent turbulence and more like constant wind shear. On the last night of another long weekend in Kingston, I washed, cut, and blow-dried my mother's lovely hair. When the combing hurt her tender scalp, she whimpered, and I reminded her how "we must suffer for beauty." We laughed the laugh we used to laugh. For a moment, on the safe island of a familiar phrase, I was fooled into thinking that I had my mother back. When we recovered from our hilarity, I helped her into her pajamas, and she said, "You are so good to do this awful thing."

"Oh, Mom," I replied, turning on the tap, "You taught me how."

I then squeezed some toothpaste on her toothbrush, panto-mimed the motions of brushing teeth, and went to turn down her bed. When I came back to the bathroom, my mother was quietly brushing her hair with her toothbrush, huge white streaks of paste smearing through her fresh new haircut.

Chapter 20.

⟨The Wrong Questions⟩

As MY MOTHER'S WORLD DIMINISHED, I had to rebuild my own. I dusted off my toolbelt and built cedar decks with a local carpenter. I began to play my flute again, and I discovered a local bar where jazz musicians invited me into their circle on Monday nights. The club became a home away from home. Then I landed my first money-making gig at the Jamestown S'Klallam Tribe teaching writing to tribal officers. Later I worked with their summer youth program and then started holding seminars at the nearby US Navy base. Anne, a local ceramic artist, had read a review I'd written of her work, and she invited me to lunch. We became fast friends.

I met a travel writer, also new in town, and we compared notes about the lives we'd left behind. He was one of the few people in town I told about Trey. Haas had impossibly long eyelashes, and his Lebanese childhood informed many of his short stories. Soon he and one of his various boyfriends were spending holidays with my family. Even for regular dinners, he always arrived with a bottle of Prosecco or, if he was feeling flush, Veuve Clicquot. He wrote for *Frommer's* travel guides and was often jetting to Dubai or the Galapagos to meet a deadline.

As my work life picked up, I registered for a Washington State Business Identification Number. Almost immediately I began to receive free promotional items: magnets, stationery, ballpoint pens. Since my business name was rather long, "Writing Seminars with Christine Hemp," the mass-mailing label invariably cut it short. One afternoon I opened my mailbox and found a bubble-wrap envelope containing yet another sample ballpoint pen. This one, glittery scarlet, was adorned with gold letters: *WRITING SEMINARS WITH CHRIST.*

Soon after receiving the pen, catalogs floated in like flotsam from Noah's flood. Church supply companies had somehow got hold of my name, and all denominations blessed me with the endless possibilities: clergy cassocks and collars, liturgical desk calendars, and one offered me a "super-spiritual-special" on altars and kneelers. I pictured Jesus standing at the $999 Oak Veneered Pulpit (available in a variety of finishes) discussing passive versus active voice, or the definite and indefinite pronoun. Of course, he'd be wearing the fashionable Cross-and-Lily chasuble (starting at $105), its gold braid glinting as he lifted his hands to talk about the power of the transitional clause. The image was prescient: mastering transitions was the skill I needed most. At the time, I believed I'd already made the biggest one of my life.

On a dark winter morning, an email from my father blew into my inbox around 6:30 a.m. with a "bing." He said he'd been awakened in the night again. "Your mom was whimpering under the bed," he wrote. When he asked her what she was doing under there, she said she was helping a little bird trying to find its mother, that it couldn't find its nest.

Dad said he'd been up at 3:00 a.m. the previous night as well, changing soiled sheets. "Before bedtime she became very angry with me for sitting out on the deck with my telescope. She exploded and said, 'What are you doing here anyway? This is MY house!! You don't belong here!' I told her, 'Okay, I'll go down to the motel and sleep there then.' What a life! Or what did Hamlet say? 'Oh, what troubled lives we lead!' Or was that Job?! Love, Fath."

It didn't seem fair that my father had to weather this gale just as he and Mom had accomplished what was intended to be a simpler life: selling the Meadowdale house, planning to hike and explore the Peninsula, inviting their many friends from Seattle to their new harbor home. Dad had raised three children, led a spiritually conscious life, wound down a successful career, and moved to a new house; but now, instead of enjoying the fruits of his labors, he joined the vast ranks of unknown soldiers who look after the sick, the dying, and the demented, forced to learn skills they'd never anticipated. Dad deserved more than this.

But what does that mean, "deserve"? Job himself certainly deserved better than a body covered with weeping boils, financial ruin, and his children slaughtered, especially after leading a creative and generous life. But he sustained disaster after disaster, until finally he rails against God with unbridled moral outrage, demanding the Creator answer the existential question of all time: "Why?!" and all the attachments to that word: "Why is there suffering??! Why me?"

Lost in his world of concepts, Job is told that he's asking the wrong question entirely. In fact, God replies from the whirlwind not with an argument (ah, the limits of logic), but with that familiar Hebraic tactic: more questions. Such as "Where were *you* when I planned the earth?…Do you give the horse his strength? Do you make him leap like a locust, snort like a blast of thunder? Do you show the hawk how to fly, stretching his wings on the wind?" Using the earthliest of images, God essentially shakes Job into a state of being rather than knowing. Apparently, there is more to life's turns than Job could ever comprehend; a simple "bad" and "good" interpretation was limiting not only to himself, but to the One who made him. According to the writer of the Book of Job (and the

Tibetan Book of the Dead, among other sacred texts), "earning" a good life means very little in the Big Picture. This story painfully reminded me that things are not always as clear as we (or some religious construct) would like them to be. My having loved Trey had shown me that.

"Dad, you really need some help," Paul said gently. He'd flown from Boston for yet another family conference. All four of us were out to lunch and trying to make a game plan. Though Dad knew he needed more than Rosemary and me looking after Mom, he was still reluctant to give up his caregiving duties. Nancy Spicer was available intermittently, but Dad did not want to rely on a friend. To relinquish control was hard for him at any time, but this was particularly difficult, especially since he knew he'd be gone for a summer trip he was planning. Dad had decided he was going to climb the highest peak in the Olympic Range, and he'd have to be away from Mom for more than a week.

"She's used to my schedule," Dad said.

"But Dad, you still need more time away," my brother urged. "Just an afternoon or two. There are caregivers besides Rosemary and Christine who can help us all."

"I feel like I'm deserting her." Dad folded his large, powerful hands on the table.

Anyone who has tended the sick knows how the caregiver can get so wrapped up in the tasks at hand that the real world recedes. Full-time dementia caregivers live in their own version of an altered universe, and it's difficult to wrest them free. "She likes to have a little glass of wine before dinner," Dad said when I came to spell him the next day. I knew this about Mom, as well as all the things Dad pointed out as if I were new to Mom's care. It made him feel more in control, but it drove me crazy. I told him everything would be fine and ushered him out the front door.

Finally, we asked my therapist, Kirk, to help us navigate this next step—opening the family to outsiders. Unlike my siblings and me, my father had never engaged in therapy. Kirk was invaluable in helping me recover from my leaving New Mexico. My brother has analyzed his own mind since he was a child. And when Rosemary was little and first beginning to read, she seemed to identify words like "anxiety" with particular relish. Since she'd only read the word silently, for years she pronounced anxiety as "*ang*shitty," an appropriate noun for the Hemp Family as we entered Kirk's office.

"Can you picture a certain kind of caregiver with your wife, Peter?" Kirk asked gently.

"Well," my father said, "it's hard to think of not taking care of her myself." Dad, in his usual affable way, was looking Kirk in the eye. As I sat there with my family—minus one important member—there was a palpable sense of betrayal. In those days, speaking behind Mom's back was as horrifying as her actual disease. It seemed sneaky and wrong. Kirk continued, "If you thought of this not as disloyalty, but an act of love and support, might that change things?"

"Well, that's another way to look at it," my father said. Kirk's Birkenstocks were clearly a minor impediment to my father's willingness to engage, but Kirk was no flake. My father was giving it the old college try. Paul scribbled notes in his ever-present notebook about whether long-term care insurance would cover in-home assistance, and Rosemary and I made plans to interview possible caregivers.

"How would it feel to do some research on memory care facilities, too?" Kirk asked. We all went silent. He told us he'd be ready to discuss that, too, when we were ready. Afterward, my father shook Kirk's hand, his tall frame dwarfing my therapist's. "Thank you for helping us," my father said with genuine relief, but it sounded as if he were thanking him for fixing our refrigerator.

Paul, Rosemary, Dad, and I each had different expectations and ways to confront Mom's situation. Paul wanted to find the safest place for her. Rosemary concentrated on the practical aspects like making schedules. Dad just needed to make it through the day. But I wanted to find my mother again, even in the wilderness of her disease. Even if, like Job, I often asked the wrong questions.

Chapter 21.

∽Summit∽

M<small>T</small>. O<small>LYMPUS</small> <small>IS</small> <small>BURIED</small> <small>IN</small> the heart of the Olympic Range, a clump of mountains that thrusts from the middle of the Olympic Peninsula. At nearly 8,000 feet, Olympus, named by the British explorer John Meares in 1778, is the tallest peak. The summit is particularly difficult because the mountain is so isolated, and, though many parties try it each year, the success rate is low, mostly because it requires a long, grueling approach. My father's desire to conquer Olympus became a major preoccupation, as if climbing that mountain would somehow reverse all he faced with Mom. The planning of the trip provided a tangible goal in his otherwise stormy daily life. Rosemary, Paul, and I worried what would happen if he didn't make it to the top. Our proud father was accustomed to success.

Dad prepared for his big ascent for more than a year. He invited my brother, Rosemary's husband Freddie, and a few experienced climber friends; he also hired a professional guide. Perhaps it took him back to his big climbing days in his thirties when he made it to the top of 14,000-foot Mt. Rainier. He'd also climbed Mt. Hood and Mt. Adams. The 1980 eruption of Mt. St. Helens had captivated him so much he'd driven miles up into the National Forest to camp on a logging road, so he could witness the terrible beauty of that mountain blowing its top. Afterward he brought me a small jar of ash.

My father sketched the mountains he could see from the condo deck, labeling the crags and shading in the valleys, but Mt. Olympus remained hidden, deep in the center of the Range. As Dad imagined his epic climb, Mom played with the dollhouse her grandfather had made her when she was a child. Dad bought her a tiny new chair and a sofa. While Mom disappeared into the world of miniature, my father mapped his route up the giant pinnacles. His face was like that range and the weather that moved across it. Sometimes it settled on his tall, handsome forehead, sometimes in the mouth, but mostly in his blue eyes, bright as glaciers.

The climbing plans kept my father going, but his daily life (and ours) was getting harder.

"I keep waiting for the women with casseroles," my sister growled as we cleaned up dinner at Mom and Dad's. We'd ushered Dad off to the stormy coast. Mom and Celia were arranging little wooden ducks in a long row across the carpet. We'd finally hired a caregiver, a woman named Lily whom Mom actually loved, but Lily only came once or twice a week, and we could no longer leave Mom alone. She'd forget the stove was on. And a neighbor had found her walking down the hill—in her signature springing step—to the ferry dock one day, smiling as if she had a mission. After that, we had to get a special lock for the door, a move that made all of us cringe.

"No, Gra'ma!! THIS way!" Celia shouted, and Mom obediently followed Celia's line of miniature ducks. Celia shouted to me, "Christine! It's actually MORE fun playing with Gra'ma now— because she forgets the rules of the games we play, and I can win every time. This pleases me greatly!"

Rosemary and I didn't dare set anything down or it would disappear. The silver serving spoons had gone missing. Dad had reported finding plates in the dresser drawers. The can opener never turned up. During the weekend we'd found Mom at the sink rinsing a huge kitchen knife under the running water, her own hand slipping down the sharp edge. Rosemary blurted, "Mom!! Be careful!" to which Mom calmly replied, "Oh, I won't cut myself; I've been doing this for years." That same afternoon Rosemary was cleaning Mom's closet of soiled clothing and I was doing laundry. From the living room, where the temperature hovered around eighty degrees as Mom inevitably cranked up the thermostat every time we turned our heads, Celia shouted, "Come on, Gra'ma! You can do it!" I rushed in to find Celia waving her arms, "We're on the big wide sea, and the coffee table is our life raft, Gra'ma! Come on! Get right up there! You can do it! We're in this togetty! We can sail togetty!" Mom lay back across the table with a smile on her face, her arms outstretched like a bird while Celia vaulted from couch to chair to couch, cheering for her brave, intrepid grandmother.

Rosemary asked me under her breath, "But where are all the older women who are supposed to take care of *us*? Where are Mom's Book Club friends?" Dad had specifically kept all their friends at bay and we missed them terribly, wishing they, too, could be a part of Mom's decline. But he would not allow his and Mom's privacy invaded, except for one caregiver, Lily, who sang to Mom in a pure contralto voice. Soothing for all of us.

"I just wish Mom and Dad's friends would storm the gates." Rosemary shut the dishwasher with a bang. I dried a big pot. Rosemary put beef stew in the freezer for Dad, and I'd made some pasta sauce for the next dinner. I spooned the leftovers from Rosemary's lamb into a plastic container.

In the living room, our aging mother's beaming face looked into Celia's, their quiet dialogue a bond as ancient as all the conversations among mothers, daughters, sisters, and granddaughters. Soon Mom was up and following us around the house again, reading aloud. This time she wasn't reading the list and calendar that Dad had left, but a quotation from Celia. Rosemary had transcribed it for her, and Mom kept copying it over and over on the ubiquitous yellow note pads. She stood in the middle of the living room, read aloud, and shaped each word of her granddaughter's language like a poem: "And the angelfish was swimming fast and glorious like a real angel…"

Suddenly Rosemary stopped putting the silver away and looked at me hard. "Christine…" I stopped midstep. "Maybe *we* are the women with the casseroles."

In August the Olympus climbing party gathered for the big ascent. Dad had brought Mom to my house, and Paul, just in from Boston, shouldered his pack then threw it in the back of Dad's Acura. They were going to pick up Rosemary's husband, Freddie, at the ferry. Dad hugged Mom, then climbed in and started the engine. Mom waved, and she and I returned to the cottage and sat on the sofa. "Well, what shall we do now?" she said.

That night Mom slept on the capacious couch, one that Dad had moved along to me from the Meadowdale house, one which they didn't need in their condo. When I retired for the night up the ladder to my tiny sleeping loft, Mom looked up and said, "Oh, so high…" I told her I'd be right up there if she needed me. In the morning, however, her confusion about being away from home was complicated by a new drug the doctor had prescribed, Aricept, which was supposed to delay the symptoms of dementia. She held her stomach and moaned in pain, her face panicked and contorted. I put the pill bottle away for good.

"All those people are going home now," she said, taking a bite of toast.

"What people, Mom?" Mom proceeded to pack and repack her suitcase as if she were leaving.

"Where's Peter?" This was probably the twentieth time that morning. "Hmmm." She dug into her suitcase. "And what time are we going home?"

Then Callie began meowing, and Badger threw up a huge hairball onto the rug. Mom began complaining about "all this stuff here," pointing to my one-room house littered with clothes, most of them hers. Scaling Mt. Olympus suddenly seemed like a lark. I wondered what had become of my Big Life? The one I thought I was going to live with the love of my life? Children? A family of my own? Was I destined only to be a parent to my aging parents and "Auntie Christine" to my nieces? The only skill I seemed to be using was improvisation, one I was also honing at the jazz nights in town. Whenever Mom got too much for me, I'd disappear into a melody in my head and finger the flute solo I might play in "Black Orpheus," which, for some reason, seemed to have become my signature tune among the jazz crowd.

"Where did you say my husband is?" Mom took one of my sweaters, folded it, and stuffed it into her suitcase.

"*Mom*, you are driving me *crazy!*" I threw down the cat-puke rag and stood up.

As if curing me of a nervous tic, my mother replied calmly, "What you've got to do is block it out. Block it *out*. After having had three children, I know how to do that."

Rosemary and Celia finally arrived a couple days later, laden with more groceries and new energy. "How about this?" Rosemary said, waving a cold bottle of Sauvignon Blanc. We three slept in the loft, as usual, while Mom snoozed on the couch with Badger and Callie. In the morning, light shone through the round window in the gable end of the cottage. "Look!" Celia said, emerging from the foggy nest of sleep, her baby cheeks still flushed, "There are the clouds! The sun rised up and then all the night light went out." Her cadences seemed to come straight from Shakespeare. Celia's love of language was actually physical. She often paced back and forth in a practice she called "Walking and Thinking," which involved interior dialogues between imaginary characters like "Mishgin" and "Jacquie." The content was impenetrable, but the nature of Celia's characters' dialogue wasn't hard to follow: an argument, an emphatic persuasion, or pure excitement. She squeezed her hands hard and clutched in the air beside her ears, her intake of breath punctuating the intensity of the narrative. Rosemary was concerned about the obsessive pacing and asked Celia's pediatrician about it, but the doctor assured her that many children with interior lives "pace." Apparently, Louisa May Alcott and Emily Dickinson both enacted their creative lives by their own equivalent of "walking and thinking." To mask her intensity, however, as an adult Alcott trained herself to clasp her hands behind her back.

As Celia walked and thinked in the tiny cottage living room and Mom asked endless questions about Dad's whereabouts, I thought about my father's interior narrative up on that mountain peak. I hoped it was meeting his expectations. But then, every trip my father took was an adventure. He had traveled around the globe more than once, one of the first members of United Airlines' Million Miler Club; he rode shotgun in an F-16 jet; and he even climbed up the tiny ladder to the tip of Seattle's Space Needle, the year they hired him to write them an ad campaign. The black-and-white photo of him in suit and tie, circa 1968, on top of that Needle shows him smiling and waving down to photographers on the observation deck.

For my seventeenth birthday, a month before I headed off to my freshman year at college, Dad took me on my first trip to New York, a destination full of history and sophistication for our West Coast family. He'd always brought back stories from business trips to Manhattan—roasted chestnuts from sidewalk vendors, the choir at the Cathedral of St. John the Divine, and skaters on the pond at Central Park. Once he brought Mom a nightie from Bonwit Teller, and the shiny lavender-flowered Bonwit's shopping bag hung on her closet doorknob for years.

On our way to New York, Dad had one business stop in Toronto. I explored the lavish hotel room and came upon a strange toilet-like piece of plumbing in the bathroom. "What's this?" I asked him, bringing him into the bathroom, "A tiny sink to wash your clothes in?"

"It's a bidet," my father told me. I heard the word as "B-Day" like a birthday. In a way it was, I suppose, because my father explained with unembarrassed authority, "Europeans use it to wash their genitals. Often before and after sexual intercourse." A wave of sexual awareness moved through my belly, and I pictured a French woman with ample breasts. Squatting? Dipping her washcloth under the faucet and then what? Where was the man during this ritual? I couldn't shake the image from my mind and was amazed that some countries provided for the luxuries of making love, a mystery that had so far eluded me.

The evening Dad and I arrived at La Guardia we discovered that two of our bags had not made it from Toronto, so we checked into the Plaza Hotel with carry-ons and only one suitcase. I was crushed because I'd packed my long coral gown, a halter dress I'd sewn myself specifically for New York. When we arrived in our room, a suite with dark oak paneling and plush velvet curtains, I was immediately distracted from my sartorial woes by a huge bouquet of flowers and a linen handkerchief in a box with a ribbon from the Plaza Hotel shop. The card was addressed to me from the manager, a business friend of my father's.

When we began dressing for dinner, I discovered another gown in the lone suitcase, a pale blue prairie dress, and a pair of platform huarache sandals, not my ideal evening-in-New-York outfit, but it would have to do.

"Is this okay?" I asked my father as I came out of the bathroom, "Mexican shoes with a linen dress?"

"You look perfect!" he said, glancing up from shining his shoes. "Beautiful!" He tightened his red-striped tie and put on his jacket. I was still mourning my lost halter dress, but once we arrived downstairs in the lobby I was too dazzled to care.

Even in the 1970s, the restaurant at the top of the St. Regis Hotel harked back to a Cary Grant movie. Pillars of marble, ornate molding, flesh-colored stucco, and pale pink tablecloths. Heavy chandeliers lit the dining room, and the tinkle of waiters crisscrossing the carpeted floors added to the air of celebration and grown-up pleasures. My father ordered a bottle of champagne, another first for me, and the evening opened up like a rose. We talked about his college days and speculated about mine to come.

"Do you think I can *do* college, Dad?" I pondered, sipping my crystal glass of bubbly.

"Of course you can!" he beamed, "You will thrive at college." He gestured briefly to the waiter that we were ready to order.

By the time the prime rib arrived I wondered if Dad knew I was looped. I had been tipsy only once, just a couple months before, at my high school graduation party. On my way to the ladies' room I could feel the boundaries of my world turn fluid. Looking in the mirror I didn't so much mind the prairie dress and felt privileged to know something I was sure the other women in the bathroom did not: the bidet.

After the plates were cleared, the orchestra struck up a tune, and my father said, "Let's dance." I clutched my dessert fork and hissed, "Daddy! Are you kidding?" All the tables were full by then, and I was horrified. Plus, what about the shoes?!

"Come on," he said, pushing his chair back and standing with his hand outstretched. My father's will be done. Fortified by champagne, I let my six-foot-four, handsome father steer me around the room, squeaky huaraches and all. Soon we were joined by other dancers; the chandeliers sparkled, and the room twirled.

When the dessert tray came around my father suggested we go have an Irish coffee in Greenwich Village. Though I'd never heard of an Irish coffee, it struck me as a wonderful idea. I knew that "The Village" was a different part of Manhattan, but I didn't know why exactly. The cab took us to a bar called Jack Delaney's. I liked the whipped cream on the drink and was careful to wipe my upper lip. When the piano started playing, I began to hum the harmony to Carole King's "It's Too Late." The player heard me and motioned for me to come over to the piano. "Go ahead," Dad said and ordered another Irish coffee. After dancing at the St. Regis, singing in a nearly empty bar was a piece of cake. I knew all the words to a Carly Simon song, too. When the player launched into "You've Got a Friend," I was really cooking, and the harmonies came easily. The player looked up at me and grinned as he sang. That's when I entered the music. I was unaware of the bar, my father, or even that I wasn't wearing the perfect dress. The piano swelled "and you need a helping hand," was perfectly in tune—or at least that's what I thought after the Irish coffee. The music and the words seemed to be married to each other, the intertwining harmonies drawn in my head, lines parallel, moving closer to, then away from, one another.

We were given gracious applause when we finished. More people had gathered in the bar, and, for a brief moment, those disparate people had become a family. The song had made it so. It wasn't until we were in the cab on our way back to the Plaza that Dad told me my piano friend was a homosexual, that his boyfriend had been sitting next to Dad at the bar, upset that he'd let me sing with his partner. Dad, in his cheerful way, had softened the partner's irritation by making it clear I was his daughter, and we all waved goodbye. This was my first encounter with the notion that artists stretch the boundaries of convention, that there were more ways to live than at home in Meadowdale. "I was so proud of you, singing up there," my father said, as the cab pulled up to the twinkling lights of the Plaza.

The next day my head hurt, and by the time we'd eaten break-fast in the Oak Room, seen the Foucault Pendulum at the United Nations, and encountered the mayhem of Wall Street, Dad noticed I was a little raggedy. The City was scrambling with life, and he steered me through the crowds. The Stock Exchange triggered a severe Not Here Feeling, and the glass windows overlooking hundreds of men yelling and waving scraps of paper sent me into a tailspin. My body lifted away from my mind, and my disorientation manifested itself in an existential blur.

At lunch I still had nausea, and New York no longer seemed twinkly and glamorous. I'd never seen a city with pavement that looked like a collage. Gum wrappers, paper cups, all kinds of trash. Women were wearing a long skirt called the "midi," where the hemline went all the way to the calf.

"Fashion starts in Paris," my father said, "then it comes to New York. It will be a while before this wave reaches the Pacific Northwest." We sat outdoors at Rockefeller Center, and Dad ordered us gazpacho. It arrived in a huge flat bowl with parsley floating on the top. The onions made my stomach turn again, and home seemed very far away. The big world wasn't "out there," but "right here." The people on the street, the newspapers, were all making noise about President Nixon's possible resignation—to avoid a trial for impeachment. Even the waiters were ranting about it. Radios blared from the storefronts.

Penn Station at rush hour was hot, ripe, and crowded. Dad posted me next to the suitcases (which had finally arrived in New York) while he went to purchase our tickets for Washington, DC I tried to look nonchalant, weight on one leg, United Airlines bag slung over one shoulder. The pressing humanity and heat, though, made me dizzy.

Tied to my island of luggage, I was helpless to fend off predators. So, when a man wearing a loose grin and a flappy raincoat moved through the throng at an odd angle, my alarm bells went off before anything strange occurred. He did not walk exactly, but veered toward me in a false swagger, his head obviously turned the other direction. But when he got within five feet of me, he looked directly at my face, opened his raincoat, unzipped his dirty brown pants, and waved a limp penis at me. Heat and horror coursed through me—my face turned hot—and I froze.

My first real thought was my dress. My spun-cotton pink shift with the nice strawberry pattern should not be seeing this. Yet I couldn't run and leave the bags. The commuters hurried to their trains without noticing a thing. Calling for help was unthinkable, as I was not being robbed or assaulted. In fact, the entire episode lasted only a matter of seconds. I turned away with the same revulsion I felt when Billy Duke threw up in front of the class in first grade, little spatters of vomit landing on my new white knee socks. In a second the man faded into the crowd.

"All aboard for Washington, DC TRACK 9. BOARDING ON TRACK 9," the loudspeaker blared through the station.

"Let's get out of this city," I said to my father who strode back waving two tickets.

"Okay! We're off!" he said with his familiar new-leg-of-a-journey bravado. He waved for a redcap, and soon we were on the train speeding south because the next day Dad had a meeting with the US Federal Energy Administration committee on tourism, to which he was appointed to by the governor of Washington State.

I kept quiet on the train, still shaken by the man in the dirty trousers. My father thought my stomach must still be a little upset and asked if I wanted the window seat. I could not tell him what had happened during our brief separation. And what words would I use exactly? Such a thing had never happened to me before, and I wondered vaguely if it might have been my fault. Had I invited this man somehow? In what strange way did it relate to the delights and possibilities of the bidet? The train hurtled south toward our nation's capital. My own confusion, however, was only part of the hubbub on the train. Conductors pressed transistor radios to their ears, and strangers were swapping opinions about the state of the presidency.

The Mayflower Hotel was abuzz with the news, too, and we hurried to our room to turn on the television. Richard Nixon's sad, loose face filled the screen. His cheeks were flushed and damp. He told us that to leave office ran against every fiber of his body. The embarrassing display rendered us mute until Dad said, "He's just down the street. He's talking right now." When Nixon finished his tearful announcement, Dad said, "Let's walk down to the White House, shall we?" Without unpacking or changing our clothes, we joined the throngs of Americans on the streets. Hecklers jeered; television cameras, like giant eyes, flashed and rose above the crowds, their lights flooding the fading summer night. A mammoth effigy of Nixon staggered by with a spike through its head. People waved signs that said WANTED and a face of Nixon under it. Hoards milled around the entrance to the gate at 1600 Pennsylvania Avenue, and, along with everyone else, we pressed in closer. A parting of the crowd revealed the White House gate swinging open, and a black stretch limo nosed out slowly. Police officers hollered, "Get back!" and the crowd fanned. Dad and I were standing within a foot or two of the car when he blurted, "Why that's Henry Kissinger!" Police lights reflected in Kissinger's glasses and his wife Nancy's white-blonde hair. Then they were gone, slithering up Pennsylvania Avenue.

The next morning my father's meeting was canceled, and we watched Nixon's last wave on television as he and his family stepped into the helicopter on the White House lawn. Then we heard a chopper overhead, and Dad pointed out the hotel window.

After Nixon's departure, Dad suggested an antidote to the hub-bub of the previous day and the presidential crisis. The Impressionist wing at the National Gallery filled me with calm. I loved the spacious rooms and couches right in front of a certain painting. I also loved how, when I squinted, Monet's pictures looked just like photographs. At lunch in the museum café, my father told me about his own painting career at the California School of Fine Arts before marriage and children nudged him into a more lucrative career in advertising. "You can be anything you want to be," he said, sipping his black coffee. "Anything."

We recounted the events of the previous days and waxed lyrical about the Plaza, dinner at the St. Regis, and Jack Delaney's. When he brought up the previous afternoon, however, my face clouded over.

"Yeah, I was glad to leave New York," I poked at my turkey sandwich.

"What was wrong at Penn Station?" Dad asked, putting his cup down. "You seemed so distracted when we got on the train. What happened?" I twirled my spoon in my chocolate mousse.

"What happened?" my father pressed.

"Well, there was a man…" I bowed my head and shook it, unable to offer one more word. Then, with the same matter-of-fact tone he'd used to explain the bidet, he said, "Did he expose himself to you or something?"

I looked up at my father in disbelief. When he saw my response, he reached right across the French rolls, dessert dishes, and gallery maps, grabbed my hand, and laughed out loud. Not in conde-scension, nor in ridicule. In one short moment, the nastiness and shame of the previous afternoon turned into filmy vapor, rising up from the table and fading like the pale clouds of Monet. When my father squeezed my hand, I laughed, too, relieved that he had now heard the worst and he was not shocked; furthermore, he'd turned the moment into something I could handle, one that would not manhandle me.

I then recounted the gory details of the man in the dirty trousers. Dad shook his head. "There are truly sick people in the world," he explained. "And I'm so sorry that happened to you. I'm just glad to know what made you so anxious; we'd had such a good time in the City." We both laughed—me with utter relief—and my father stood, slapped his pockets, and said, "Whaddya say we go see the Tomb of the Unknown Soldier?"

To celebrate the men emerging from their seven-day trek in the wilderness, Rosemary and I made a big chicken dinner. The car rolled up to the cottage, and Celia shouted "Grandfather!" Paul and Freddie tumbled out, dusty and smiling. Mom said, "Oh!" and ran down the steps toward Dad, who opened the driver's door and slowly unfolded his six-foot-four frame from the car.

"Mary," he said, nearly in tears, hugging her close. For a moment there was no Alzheimer's, no Olympus peak, no linear time and space. Dad's hand stroked Mom's head against his shoulder, and the embrace briefly reassured me of Dad's certain success, the stability of my parents, the order of things.

I searched Dad's sunburned face for signs of "summit." Instead of inquiring, though, I blurted, "Did you guys see Mom, Rosemary, Celia, and me waving from the beach?" As if, at that elevation, they could have spotted us. My father's face beamed, and my heart raced. He'd made it. Yes, my father must have made it to the top of that mountain.

"Paul and Freddie made it!" my father boomed. Rosemary and I exchanged a quick glance. The moat of cheer was one of my father's greatest defense mechanisms. "And only three in the whole party actually made it to the summit, the other being Jim's wife Kathy!" My father held out his arm proudly toward Paul and Freddie.

We all filed in for dinner, the boys stiff and hungry. During the meal Paul explained how Dad had made it all the way to the glacier field just before the final ascent.

"It was really a tough climb," Paul said, reaching for more potatoes to pile on his plate. Freddie described with care the steep rocks and the vertiginous view as Dad listened, too, quietly downing another glass of wine.

"I was really nervous there, toward the end," Paul admitted, buttering some of Rosemary's homemade bread. "I almost didn't make that last scramble."

As Freddie described the long, three-day haul to base camp, my father's face looked like a map of intersecting trails. His blue eyes glittered when Freddie spoke of the summit, but his cheeks drooped when the story got to the part where he turned back. His cheekbones were even more pronounced with the sunburn and the loss of a few pounds.

"Like any good climber," Freddie said, respectfully glancing over at my father, "he didn't want to hold everyone back. So at the glacier field below the final ascent, he decided to return to camp." Dad's face grew suddenly inscrutable, his eyes focused on something I couldn't see. Mom, however, gleamed as she took another bite of green beans, the conversation flowing over her like a mountain rivulet.

Then Paul helped himself to more chicken and skimmed over the summiting part of the story. "On the descent we were pretty worn out. Truly." My brother looked up. "But when we arrived at the meadow at the edge of the glacier, a half-day's hike above base camp, we spotted someone standing there in the evening light. Waiting for us." Paul wiped his mouth with his napkin. The sun, setting over the Straits, slanted into my little cottage and splashed orange gleams across the wall.

"It was Dad," Paul said. "He'd hiked all the way back up there to welcome us, to bring us roast beef sandwiches."

Chapter 22.

⮊ Body Memory ⮈

MY INTIMATE CONVERSATIONS WITH BUDDY addressed things important to us both. I needed connection, and he needed clarity. To get that connection, I found that the more I treated Buddy honestly—even clucking to him if he gave me a rude face—the more supple and engaged he became. When I asked him with firm body energy to move over when I was cleaning his feet, or not to nibble at my sleeve, Buddy actually paid more attention to me, not less. And then he offered things I didn't ask, too, like lowering his head and willingly poking his nose into the halter. Finding me instead of me trying to find him.

Ken had taught me that this wasn't some secret "horse-whispering" code known only to a precious few. This was available to everyone, but it required holding one's own self accountable. I needed to take stock of my own motives as well as being sensitive to how Buddy was feeling.

Not exactly easy, no matter how good the words sound. Sometimes words just got in the way of this difficult art because it wasn't about my language at all; it was about Buddy's.

In the early spring Ken and I are still working on "bit issues." Buddy is chomping and pushing against the bit while I try to keep him at a quiet walk. He isn't giving his jaw and softening at the poll, the bendable place where a horse's head meets its neck. As Ken is showing me, Buddy just wants to get away from that thing in his mouth, and he isn't thinking about much else, least of all the woman on his back.

"He's just hitting up against a wall of resistance," Ken says from the middle of the ring. "He's not listening to your leg. He's only involved with the bit right now—and the inconvenience of it all." The sun pokes through the clouds and then disappears. As I ride Buddy around the ring, his mouth feels hard and unresponsive.

Ken tightens the scarf around his neck. "Pay attention to that resistance," he says. "This is extremely important to Buddy, so you need to talk to him about it. It's a conversation worth having. It's real and it's happening now." Buddy throws up his head. "See? He's bracing, because you're taking away his protective devices—you're telling him that it's not cool for him to throw his head and ignore you. That's scary for him. The tiny contact you're asking is like saying, 'Yes, I hear that you don't like that, but what about this instead?'"

My contact with Buddy's mouth gives in for a split second, and, instead of loosening the reins completely, I yield to his momentary softness but keep a quiet connection.

Ken walks along with us about six feet away. "You're doing this to let him know that he doesn't *have* to brace in order to feel okay about himself, that it's actually easier to give in the mouth, the poll, and his whole body will be more comfortable."

It is hard to see Buddy in discomfort, though.

As if reading my thoughts, Ken says, "You have to wade through the crap and climb out the other side of this stuff." I think of all the wading I'd done in recent years and wonder whether I have climbed out the other side. Working with Buddy seems to bring it all back again. The disaster in Riojos and others that followed so quickly upon its heels. My island of home had turned out so much different from what I'd expected. And now Buddy was teaching me that I have *more* work to do. It never seems to be over.

"If he were a very young horse," Ken says, "you wouldn't have to do a lot of this, really. You would have raised him by offering the best deal already. He would have trusted people more. He would have felt secure. But he's carrying a lot of habits and protection techniques from a time before you. You can't take that personally."

I urge Buddy on gently with my leg, then release so he can step forward. With that release immediately he begins listening. He moves into a nice swinging walk, moving with his whole body, not just his brain. He isn't even thinking about the bit. One ear cocked back toward me, his mouth softens, the reins give slightly in my hands—as if he's giving back what I'm giving him.

"See?" Ken says, smiling under the brim of his hat, then walks over to where Buddy and I come to an easy stop. "Sometimes we just have to look *past* the pain. Just so that you can let them know it doesn't have to be painful *now*. Okay, let him rest." Buddy stands quietly and yawns.

"Now. Ask him to go out on the rail again. Let him know you want to go somewhere." With an opening of my leg, Buddy moves out, his hind end propelling us forward gracefully. "Okay, good," Ken says. "Now release all mental and physical intention of forward. Be a sack of potatoes on top of him."

"What?" I ask, wondering why I'd let Buddy just go on his own without any direction.

"Do it!" Ken says, so I let my body and hands go limp and vague.

Immediately Buddy stops. No pulling of the reins, just the absence of my mental intention is reflected in his body.

"He's getting there!" Ken relaxes against the fence rail and waves his right hand in the air. "He's really starting to listen to you. He knew you weren't asking anything of him right there. He stopped of his own accord. Someday all you'll have to do is *think* "stop" or "turn right" or "canter." It won't be mechanical, it will be intuitive. See? There's your lick and chew."

Ken always ends a lesson when the horse has a success, something to be proud of. Buddy and I both feel it. The wind picks up, and Ken takes his keys out of his pocket to get ready to go. He heads toward his truck, then turns back. A gust of wind picks up his hat, and he crushes it down on his head. "It's just as important for Buddy to know when you're *not* asking something of him. You're helping his body memory find a new path."

Sometimes it is hard to believe I am helping Buddy. There is so much to learn. But of one thing I am certain: Buddy is helping me.

Chapter 23.

∽The Optimist's Daughter∽

As Mom's condition went downhill, Dad became more and more grateful for Rosemary and me spelling him for a night or two. Often he'd drive the three-and-a-half hours to the coast and loved staying at the Kalaloch Lodge in Olympic National Park. Robust at 74, he hiked the long ocean beaches and ended his day with a martini or two and a good dinner. The historic inn was up to his standards, and it was also far away from his wife's problems.

One evening when I was staying with Mom, the PBS News Hour aired a tribute to Eudora Welty, who had just died at the age of 92. Serving our dinner at the coffee table, I reminded Mom that Welty was among her top favorite writers. The familiar spines of *Losing Battles* and *The Ponder Heart* were emblems of Mom's rich interior life. Her face clouded, though, when I mentioned these titles. She said she thought she recognized the author's name but could not remember her stories. The commentator read a line from *The Optimist's Daughter*: "Life is nothing but the continuity of its love." Mom's eyes filled with tears.

I, too, seemed to be the optimist's daughter, always turning the coin to find the brighter side as my mother always had, and continued to do so even in her disease. When I mentioned the events that had brought me home from Riojos, for example, she looked at me quizzically. I gave her some handholds like mentioning my ex. Mom said, "Now who was Trey again?"

"*Mom*," I said, "leaving Trey was one of the most traumatic moments of my life!" She promptly replied. "Well, it's a good thing I've forgotten him then, isn't it?"

Mom had always protected us from the malignant forces of this world. I pondered whether this was why I'd been so unprepared for Trey's cruelty. I didn't think I was a naive person. And the men in my life, including boyfriends, had all been such decent people—so why hadn't I seen it coming? Or had I pushed it aside, fanning my own dreams? Now Mom's disease was beginning to eat away at my bright-penny resolve. If one abandons unadulterated optimism, does that automatically render you a pessimist?

After listening to the Welty quotation on TV, Mom got quiet and said, "You know, when you're this age, you think about your life and wonder if you've done the right things..." She sniffled a bit and I was surprised at her lucidity, Welty's words having reached her through the gauze around the once-rich library of her brain.

"Mom, you *have* done the right things. You made the best family ever." I picked up her napkin and a piece of chicken that had fallen to the floor.

"But I loved you children, I loved you," she said, justifying something I couldn't figure out. Her voice wavered.

Groping to make some sense of this strange chapter in my mother's story, I thought of my own. Trey had actually given me a new muscle for rowing through sorrow. I also wondered if maybe Mom's life's work, nourishing us and making us feel loved and safe in the world, was in preparation for her own bumpy ride at the end. For who but someone loved deeply would attend to the reckless lunacy of this disease? The commentator ended the PBS tribute with another line of Welty's from *One Writer's Beginnings*: "As you have seen, I am a writer who came of a sheltered life. A sheltered life can be a daring life as well. For all serious daring starts from within."

Stuck in the lower-left corner of a framed ink drawing in the Hemp family kitchen in Meadowdale was a scrap of paper quoting J. D. Salinger's *Franny and Zooey*. It's the part where Zooey's older brother instructs him in coping with the fakery of the world. And how in the end, he says, we just have to be kind and courteous to one another. Long before we children had read this book, we knew it was important because Mom had copied it in her slanty, thin-looped handwriting. "J. D. Salinger doesn't use devout or holy lan-guage," she told us, "but he's probably one of the most religious—or spiritual—writers I've ever read." My mother especially loved the scene where Seymour Glass claims to have seen Jesus in the ashtray of a New York City taxicab.

As Mom's dementia advanced, I discovered that a taxi ashtray was as good a place as any to find solace. I cleaned up another pile of underpants my mother had stuffed into the toilet and tried to sort out this new phase in her life. And mine. None of it seemed fair. Once in college when I was outraged because my boyfriend didn't get the philosophy department job he'd applied for (his best friend with fewer credentials did), my mom had said, "Well, life is never *fair*, Christine."

But when you come from a family for whom fairness is high on the list, don't you expect the world to follow suit—at least a little? I can still hear Mom scolding when one of us hogged too many cookies or the whole box of Quisp cereal. "Don't lay your ears back!" she said, describing perfectly how horses charge with mad faces toward the bucket of grain or fresh pile of hay.

As I got older, my friends wanted to be part of my family, too. When Peggy and I met in our thirties in Boston, she told me about the rough time she'd had with her parents. I wondered how she

could possibly be attracted to my white-bread family, since her
upbringing seemed so much more glamorous. Her father was a
writer, and they'd traveled on ships to Europe. When she met my
mother and father, she said she wanted to become an honorary
member of *my* family.

One spring day she called and begged me to join her for Easter
brunch. "My Dad's going to be in town," she said gloomily. "And
his new young wife. I need fortification."

Peggy and I had become friends at Emmanuel Episcopal
Church on Newbury Street. She was a graduate student at
Harvard Divinity School and often helped served communion
after the weekly Bach cantata. The parish swelled with a consid-
erable gay and artist contingent, many homeless members, a few
Boston bluebloods, and myriad others "with a rattle," as our friend
Christopher described us. We all seemed to have arrived with a
specific longing. Outside the chapel door a banner waved in the
sun: You Are Welcome Here as Long as Your Integrity
Permits.

"Pleeeeease?" Peggy joked over the phone. "I'll give you a marble from my marble jar if you come."

When I hung up, I called my mother immediately.

"Mom, guess who I'm spending Easter with?"

When Peggy introduced me to her father outside after the Easter
service, I looked him in the eye as my own father had taught me.
"How do you do, Mr. Salinger?" and offered him a firm Peter Hemp
handshake.

Peggy's father pumped my hand. "Very well, Christine!" he
said cheerfully. "Call me Jerry." I liked him immediately. His eyes
were clear and curious, outward-looking rather than broody, as I'd
expected. At seventy he had a full head of white hair and the tall,
lanky, good looks of a tennis player. He wore a pin-striped shirt,

a green sweater vest, and a blue blazer, wool trousers, and suede bucks. He embodied charm in a natty, prep-school way, a breed of man now nearly extinct.

Peggy's father was enthusiastic about the service ("Peggy in a robe!") and the Reverend Al Kershaw's sermon. Jerry told us he was once baptized "years ago!" at a Pentecostal Church in New York. Thinking of the famous author in a fundamentalist church struck me as cognitive dissonance, but we stepped cheerily into the Public Garden on our way to the restaurant. He seemed perfectly at home in the day. I didn't perceive any grouchiness nor was he pretentious or poet-y. In fact, he was the kind of man my parents would have liked.

Tulips were bursting red and yellow, and a little wind fluttered the surface of the pond. "Is there any speaking in tongues at your church?" Jerry asked. Peggy and I laughed out loud. "No!" she said, as we passed the magnificent statue of George Washington on his swishy half-Arabian war horse. I could almost hear Holden Caulfield saying, "Old George, there."

Colleen, Salinger's young wife, giggled about the speaking in tongues. She was a nurse, and, at twenty-six, with Irish freckles and pink cheeks, she actually looked sixteen. Her plain little skirt and jacket reminded me of a Catholic uniform. ("The eternal virgin!" Peggy had told me.) I wondered how I was going to navigate these invisible family undercurrents.

"You two look like schoolgirls in your flowery dresses," Jerry said to Peggy and me. I could tell this both delighted and repulsed my friend, though she was beautiful no matter what she wore, with her long, black hair and tall, slim figure. Today she played the role of blushing daughter. I wondered again why she'd chosen me to meet her famous, reclusive father—especially when I'd overheard Christopher describe me to his new boyfriend: "Christine? Oh, she has no story. She's just an Episcopalian girl from Edmonds, Washington." Though I knew he'd said it with irony, his comment stung.

At Maison Robert, then one of Boston's ritziest restaurants, Peggy, her father, Colleen, and I were seated at a table covered with white linen and immediately served a basket of hot rolls. Peggy had told me her dad was very fussy about what he ate. I ordered soup. I figured it would alleviate any concern about getting a piece of grilled prawn stuck in my teeth. From my chair I could see beyond Jerry's shoulder to King's Chapel graveyard, one of the city's oldest burial grounds, where slate gravestones rose out of the grass like Necco candies. I carefully sipped my asparagus soup, hoping I would not implode with all the stimuli. I wished my mother were at the next table.

"But what do you do?" Jerry asked, and I was startled back to the table. I explained my patchwork jobs—teaching part-time; two nights a week doing paralegal work at a corporate law firm; and visiting Massachusetts public schools as part of their artists-in-residence program. "It's a pretty busy schedule," I said and laughed. I was too shy to talk about my writing—it felt pretentious to tell *anyone* I was an aspiring poet (much less J. D. Salinger). Jerry nodded vigorously, smiling. Peggy had told me that when she was a child she was never allowed in her father's studio except to deliver lunch to his door. I did not tell him that the space I'd found had changed my life. Instead I described the view of Boston Harbor from my loft and how at night fifty mail trucks lined up like Matchbox toys in the municipal parking lot below.

"Terrific!" he said, taking another bite of a roll and stuffing another in his jacket pocket.

It was really hard, though, in this setting not to ask The Question poised to burst from my mouth, bits of asparagus and walnuts spewing out with it. I sealed my lips to prevent it from escaping: "But Jerry! Are you still writing—or WHAT?! Will there be more stories???" My heart rate ramped up just thinking about that question hovering on my tongue. I calmed myself by thinking of my mother. Already I was memorizing the details of this lunch for her:

the easy cadences of Salinger's speech, how he loved to make soups, and his almost fanatical interest in my night job. It was the job I never wanted to talk about—proofing legal documents from 5:00 p.m. till midnight, the cash crop that kept me in groceries.

"What do you do there?" he pressed, reaching out for another roll. I recalled reading that he was in the middle of a lawsuit about some unauthorized biography. So I told him about the time the firm had flown me to Orlando to deliver a tender offer to a publishing company, how I'd had to demand to see the CEO and get the document signed, sworn to secrecy until it hit the papers the next day. Jerry was delighted.

"And what about your work with children?" I flashed on a scene in *Raise High the Roof Beam, Carpenters* where Seymour sees a stigmata on his hand after touching the heads of his baby brother and sister. I told Jerry about the previous week when I'd asked fourth-graders to bring in a special object to write about. Andrew, a child who rarely spoke, brought his father's huge wristwatch. Even in fourth grade Andrew could barely write, but when he did, the poem was about time and how his father had none for him. Our table at Maison Robert grew uncomfortably quiet. Colleen, like an eager granddaughter, dutifully wiped up the crumbs around Jerry's plate. Jerry cleared his throat and mentioned he was off to London soon. Peggy and I had both lived in London, so we chimed in simultaneously, asking what the trip was about.

"An old friend of mine is turning seventy," Jerry adjusted himself in his chair, his tall frame at home in space. "I haven't seen him for fifty years! I knew him the year I spent in Vienna. Before we grew up. Before the war. We played together—really *played*—with a vitality that is rare at any age."

"Wow," I said, imagining him as a young man, wondering what *play* meant to him. Drinking wildly? Womanizing? "It must be wonderful to have friends that long," I suggested. Out of nowhere he revealed a slice of the crankiness Peggy had told me about. His mood, like the sun leaving the graveyard out the window, turned gloomy.

"I've managed to lose most of my friends anyway," he growled, adjusting his shirt sleeve. "My friends at the *New Yorker* are all gone, and most of the others are either dead or have disappeared." He held up his half-eaten roll and addressed Colleen, "Why can't we get bread like this in New Hampshire?!" Both Peggy and Colleen betrayed a minimal cringe.

The story of Job from that morning's sermon was still in my head. Our rector, Al Kershaw, had gracefully connected Job's questions to our own, and Al read from the new translation by the poet Stephen Mitchell. I'd been mesmerized, especially about the part when God couldn't seem to answer for the problems Job endured. He just responded to Job with more questions, a new concept for me. Literature, it seems, does not solve things; it merely holds up the mirror.

As I sat there with a man whose stories dripped with kindness and compassion, I began to suspect that making something complex and beautiful isn't always in keeping with the maker. If so, would that apply to the Great Creator as well? Maybe the qualities we love in art and literature are the very things the Maker is striving for, too.

When the conversation turned to movies, Jerry was all affability. He and Colleen watched a lot of them, he said, and turned to me. "What's your favorite?" A window shade dropped in my head. Clearly a *Stormy, Misty's Foal* moment. Suddenly I blurted out "*The Red Shoes!*" the 1948 classic with Moira Shearer and Anton Walbrook, a movie long before my time, but one I'd discovered on late-night television in my teens. When Jerry said, "Yes! Yes! A wonderful film," Peggy smiled, proud that I'd passed some test.

"Did you know that *The Red Shoes* was the last Technicolor film to be made in this country?" Jerry pushed his plate away and a waiter floated by to remove it.

"No!" I said, a little too enthusiastically.

"The rights were sold to the Japanese. That's why we no longer see color like that anymore." I pictured the crimson shoes that Moira Shearer danced in until she dropped. And then I remembered the deep, red hues in our old Hemp family photo albums. Me with Lightfoot in the Fourth of July parade. Rosemary holding one of our hens, Paul and Dad stacking the firewood pile. And Mom, smiling. How strange to lose an entire range of coloration, as if the way we see the world can be erased and replaced with a new tint, a different value, though the shapes remain the same. On that afternoon in Boston I could not imagine my life's colors any different from that moment, all possibility stretching out in front of me, graceful as the swan boats on the Boston Common. My parents were happy, still young and vibrant. I felt safe in the knowledge of being loved. And, of course, my father could never have written what Peggy's father had—who could have?—but I would never trade him in. All I could see was that cracked family photo taken by a neighbor, "The five original Hemps!" my father saying, as we scrunched together in front of our shiny red Buick.

I couldn't wait to get back to my apartment and call my mother.

Chapter 24.

~Hobbled~

BUDDY OFFERED ME PLEASURES I'D put aside for years. The smell of leather, horse sweat, and hay. Riding bareback. Rubbing my hand down a sleek foreleg. The comforting sound of a horse munching at night. Picking up manure with a fork and tossing it into the wheelbarrow with a satisfying thunk. The thrilling whinny when he saw me coming up to the meadow. Such delights I'd believed were lost to me, relegated only to the memory bank or a trust fund not to be drawn upon, only passed down.

I'd even catch myself occasionally calling Buddy "Lightfoot." Buddy made time shrink. Wasn't it just the day before yesterday I was fourteen and heading off on a horse camping trip with Joanie O'Neill? That summer she invited me and a few 4-H pals on a pack trip in the mountains. Her dad drove the huge trailer filled with our horses, and we headed toward the North Cascades, where my family hiked every summer, Dad patting the huge hemlocks along the trail, saying, "This tree was here when Columbus came to America!" In fact, Joanie and I were going to the mountain valley near where Mom and Dad had been hiking on the day before I was born.

Joanie's little pinto, Flash, was Lightfoot's familiar companion, and we galloped together through the alpine meadows. Boppa had given me his old hobbles for the trip, a device used by cowboys and trail riders alike to keep a horse near camp. Usually it's two pieces of leather secured between a horse's front feet so they can walk easily, but if they try to run, they have to gallump like rocking horses and it's slow going. Most horse prefer to graze and don't stray far.

The evening after our big trek up into the high country, back at camp I hobbled Lightfoot, put a bell on him, and turned him loose with the herd. As I fell asleep to the tinkling of the bells, I felt about as close to Will James as ever, my sleeping bag my bedroll, the campfire crackling and making shadows in the night.

The next morning, I woke to someone saying, "Where's Lightfoot?" I leapt out of my dew-drenched sleeping bag, pulling on a boot, hopping on one foot to get the other one on. Sure enough that dappled gray hide was nowhere to be seen. My heart flew into overdrive. "Lightfooooooooooooooot!" I called, knowing from my family hikes how quickly the wilderness can swallow you up. My father always told us to keep to the trail. "Mountains don't care," my mother said as she stopped to touch a massive granite stone above the scree in Gothic Basin. I pictured Lightfoot in that faraway place above tree line, lost without water.

I grabbed a lead rope and hightailed it out past the other tinkling horses in the meadow, pressed my index and middle fingers to my mouth, letting out a long Frank Melang whistle. No answer. No thunder of hooves. The rising sun filtered through the trees, and I told myself to stay calm. My Levis were soaked. Spiderwebs laden with dew droplets bobbled as I swished through the vast meadow and headed up toward the forest. Above me glacier fields sparkled. In the far distance I could hear Joanie and my friends calling Lightfoot's name.

The grass was almost waist-high as I worked my way through a draw. When I came around a stand of trees, I whistled again. In an instant a white face popped its head up from the grass. "Lightfoot!!" I shouted with relief. "Lightfoot! Where have you been?" He whinnied, then ambled toward me, puzzled by my urgency, dragging the broken hobbles. He came straight over for a nuzzle. Behind him swaggered a fat little pony with mangy hair, a pal he'd befriended in the night. I threw my arms around his neck and clipped the lead rope onto his halter. We slowly returned to camp, my elegant gray gelding and the plump pony bringing up the rear. We were greeted with hot chocolate and cheers from Joanie, her mom and dad, and my friends. Sometimes what we believe to be lost forever is merely obscured by a stand of hemlock.

Chapter 25.

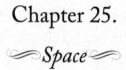

Space

To FALL IN LOVE WITH a horse, really, is to fall in love with its body. The visual beauty alone is exhilarating, but it isn't until we mingle our smells and our touch that a deepening comes into play.

I often wonder if, as in human love, we are attracted to those who appeal to our own personal tastes—literally. Our senses reveal things to us we don't think about, but we surely feel. Though I'd always done some heavy eye-rolling about those horse-crazy girls of my youth, I did notice that now when Buddy trotted up to me in the meadow my heart would lift; I felt a flow in my own flesh. This was not made up; it was real. Oh, I admired his naturally pleasing proportions and his fabulous alert ears and the whole package of his Arabian self, but when I touched his hide and ran my hand over his haunches, I began to learn his body. I came to know where he flinched (his belly) what made him feel happy (scratching his chest) and where, if I laid my hand on his forehead like a benediction, I could feel him breathe out and relax. Coming to know his body was leading me to his mind, his spirit.

Invariably, there's that nudge-nudge-wink-wink comment people make about "girls and horses!" but I wonder if, with a horse, a girl can come to understand what it means to become one with another body—without the predatory ingredient of many first sexual experiences.

In October, Ken comes to give me a lesson and Buddy, loose and grazing in the round pen, sees Ken and lifts his head, a hunk of grass hanging out of his mouth midchew. Ken pauses before walking up to him, and I notice the slight give in Buddy when Ken steps back. When Ken gives Buddy the space, Buddy perks up his ears as if to say, "Thank you!" and actually offers a step toward Ken.

"Look at that," I say.

"He's just appreciating that I didn't barge in," Ken says, pausing another beat and then putting out his hand for Buddy's nose to greet him. "There's no reason to force. He's so sensitive he can feel me from a long way off." The sun shines on Buddy's coat, and his intelligent eyes seem to take in everything. Inwardly I swoon, not wanting to admit to Ken my hopeless crush. Sometimes I can barely keep my hands off this horse, and yet Ken holds his own hands away until Buddy is ready. It isn't just timing, it's feel.

"I'm often surprised," Ken says, lighting up a smoke, "when it comes to being respectful of a horse's space. You'd think it would be women who would know about such things." Ken shakes his head laughing. "But it's the girls who want to molest their horses, plunder them with unwanted petting and kisses." Buddy noses toward me, his whiskers barely touching the back of my hand. A rush of delight courses up my forearms.

"Horses don't want to be touched all the time." Ken gently taps his cigarette, and a piece of ash falls on the dirt. "It's uncomfortable for them. I cannot understand why people pat their horses with big, heavy slaps as if they're bags of grain. For a horse—who can flick off the tiniest mosquito with his skin—that's like shouting. A horse communicates differently. They have that invisible bubble, their sensory radar."

"But what about once they let you in?" I ask, hoping Ken won't think I am one of those invasive women, unconscious of my horse's needs.

"If a horse trusts you," Ken says, "you can do just about anything with him. Clean his sheath, touch his ears, crawl under his belly. But until then, there is always wariness, even if he's standing stock-still. And any time there's tension or worry in the horse, there's danger for you. I always tell my clients to be careful, not to assume your horse is bombproof just because you love him. And every horse has a threshold. It's up to us to find out where that is—and to honor it."

I refrain from burying my nose in Buddy's sleek neck as he leans in to pull the red handkerchief from my vest pocket and waves it in the air like a magician. Ken lifts his right hand, his square fingers barely touching Buddy's forehead. Buddy drops the handkerchief into my hand and releases a long sigh, his out-breath making space for all three of us. It had been a long time since I'd known a horse this intimately. Buddy cantered right into the center of my life. As with all those we love, already it was difficult to imagine a time without him.

Chapter 26.

ᵫ *Strong and Supple Wood* ᵫ

MY QUIET, SLIM NEIGHBOR SERVED me a steaming cup of coffee and passed the half-and-half carton across his small, wooden table. Ole (pronounced "Ula") lived just a stone's throw from my beach cottage, but I had never seen his face until a couple weeks before. A friend had been over getting details about cat-sitting. I was headed out the next day on a two-week teaching gig in Maine. When Russell spotted Ole walking toward the beach, he called him over to say hi. The three of us ended up having a beer on my deck, the sun setting in streamers over the Straits.

The day after I'd returned from Maine, Ole invited me for pancakes. "My specialty," he said on the phone. I couldn't recall ever having been asked on a date for pancakes, but I agreed to come, especially since he was cooking. After so much caregiving with Mom, I was happy to have someone else make a meal, even if it was breakfast. We slowly finished our pancakes, complete with yogurt, raisins, and bananas. "It's the Norwegian way," he said, smoothing back his dark hair thick as a brush.

In the few years since leaving Riojos I'd had a brief affair with the deck-building carpenter whose kindness helped to mend my spirit. I'd dallied with a skipper of a sailing yacht, and I'd had a fling with one or two musicians. But nothing had stuck.

"So what about that fly rod?" I said to Ole, pointing to the rod mounted on a low beam.

"Oh, I used to be a fly-fishing guide in Alaska. But I really don't fish now." He followed my gaze up to the beam.

"You gave up fly-fishing? Really?"

Talking about fishing felt like talking about a lost love. I had fished very little since I'd left Riojos, and I sorely missed those mountain streams of the Southwest.

"Oh, my dad made sure I knew how to fly-fish." Ole pushed the dirty dishes aside. "He'd wake me at dawn, and we'd go steelhead-ing. After so many years, I realized that I didn't want to fish any-more." He waved away more of my questions and leaned way back on his chair, balancing with his long legs.

"But I'd like to see that fly rod," I said, amazed that anyone could just *give up* fishing. I'd been so homesick for my Sangre de Cristo rivers that even a retired rod was cause for reverence. Ole set the chair back down on all fours, cleared the plates, then reached up with both hands to lift the rod off the nails. The back of his shirt came untucked, and his jeans hung from his slender hips in a dis-turbingly appealing way.

"Okay, let's go catfishing," he said, heading out into his garden filled with hollyhocks, delphinium, Shasta daisies, and sunflowers. The door of his tiny shop was open, and little woodworking planes and odd-shaped clamps lay scattered on his tool bench.

"Catfishing?" Surely this man knew there were no catfish around here. Sea-run cutthroat and salmon, yes, but catfish?

"Any gerund in a storm," Ole said and tied a tiny piece of cloth onto the end of the tippet. His two cats, Dogger and Lorus, both dark-haired like Ole, perked up when they saw the rod jiggle. Soon they pranced and hovered, wiggled and pounced while Ole's cast landed perfectly on a tail or in front of a whisker. We laughed at the air-springs and scamperings. I silently admired the skillful back cast, his double-haul, and the gentle way his wrist stayed steady while the line made easy *S*'s in the air.

He told me he'd been born the year before me, north of the Arctic Circle, though he looked more Spaniard than Scandinavian. His parents had moved to America when he was a boy, but he still spoke the language and returned many times to Norway. His hair stuck out every which way from his head. His hazel eyes contained more than they gave away. Long pauses in our conversation stretched out like his cast. This man is *too* quiet, I thought. Not really *glittery* enough. I quickly tallied the cons on my familiar ledger, although I liked the sense of calm I felt in his presence. I sat down on his picnic bench and absorbed the sunny spring morning, flowers exploding and the cats dancing. Though he lived only two blocks from my own little house, his garden was toasty warm. Unlike my deck, where the westerlies blew mercilessly off the Straits even in summer, his garden was protected, and the temperature was ten degrees warmer than at the beach.

Ole cast a double-haul far over the delphiniums, and the cats raced to catch it. He moved elegantly through space, and his hands were alive, as if made specifically for his profession: he was a maker of bows for stringed instruments. I'd known a few luthiers but had never thought about the makers of the bows for violins, violas, or cellos. Ole told me that the bows were fashioned from a rare Brazilian hardwood called Pernambuco, once used predominantly in Europe for dying fabrics. When mixed with water, the dust from the wood turns a purplish red. Apparently in the nineteenth century the French discovered that this strong and supple wood had another purpose, and they created what we now know as the modern bow.

"I heard you on NPR, the piece about your poem in space," Ole said, changing the subject and breaking the cat-fishing spell. "It must be great to have your poem up there. Would you read me that essay and poem sometime?"

"Oh," I said, surprised at his non sequitur, "sure." (What writer would not fling herself onto the ground and grab the pant leg of anyone who requested such a thing?) Then he suggested we go see the local jazz combo the next night.

"I was given some tickets today. Shouldn't go to waste. But I don't have a car," he said. "Would you mind meeting me there?" I found the timing of the invitation a little off, asking me on one date so quickly upon the heels of this one. We'd hardly digested our pancakes, but I agreed. I had no other plans. And the combo included several musician friends.

Before the jazz, I met him for a beer at a bar that looks over the bay. We sat in the sunshine and he admired my earrings. Made by a friend, they were pale-green beach glass laced with silver. When he lifted his hand, reached over the beers, and touched the right earring, I blushed. A delicate sensation ran through his fingers into the earring, down my earlobe, and into my belly. Flustered, I said, "Well, shall we go hear the music?"

The combo was terrific—no need for talking—and afterward we loaded his bike onto the bike rack of my car, and I drove us back to the beach in silence. Clearly, conversation wasn't Ole's strong point. As a rule, the Hemp Family was never without comments about even the smallest of minutiae. A running joke when we wanted even more detail was "What color were the bathroom tiles?"

I was baffled by, and a little uncomfortable with, those who were at ease with wordlessness. What shaped this man's thoughts if there were no words? I was used to banter, quick give-and-take. Parry and pounce. Ole did not participate in such a dance. As I pulled my car into his driveway where Lorus and Dogger waited, their bright cat eyes shining in the headlights, I resorted to a Hemp Family line, one always delivered with complete irony, "So!" I said, channeling my father's booming voice, "Have we said everything there is that needs to be said?"

Ole shook his head in disbelief, got out of the car, removed his bike, followed his cats through the gate, and waved goodbye.

When I called Rosemary to tell her about my quiet Bowmaker, she reported that Celia, too, had had some boy encounters. "What?" I said, incredulous. I pictured Celia in the new vest I'd sewn for her first day of kindergarten. The blue cotton fabric, splashed with yellow, red, and green stars all over it, definitely made a statement. I'd lined it with red silk (her favorite color) and had chosen buttons carved with little clocks. Time and space. Fitting attire, I thought, for Albert Einstein Elementary School.

"Apparently her friend Josh wants to hug her all the time," Rosemary said. I could hear my sister stirring a pan on the stove. "It's both fascinating and repellent to her, I think," Rosemary said.

A day or two went by. Rosemary and I couldn't see a problem with Josh's hugging, but soon we kept hearing that Josh—another man of few words—scooted very close to her on the school bus and even wanted to kiss her (something I'd yet to experience with the Bowmaker).

"I told Celia that she could say 'no,'" Rosemary told me. Understandably, Josh's overtures got tiresome, especially when Celia reported how Josh tried to get her attention. "He licks the bottom of his shoes!" All I could think of was Mom's familiar dictum, "Men: They have gaps."

Several days later when Celia got off the bus, the story had shifted slightly. "Well it was a Bug Day...," Celia had said (her interpretation of "Big Day"). "I'm NOT going to marry Josh after all." These nuptial plans were news to us all, but the update was no less a relief.

"Why not?" Rosemary had asked casually, grabbing Celia's hand to walk her home. As if commenting on the weather, Celia replied, "Oh, he's feeding on those other girls, munching on those other feasts."

Soon after the pancake feast, I flew to Southern France with Sas. We'd conjured up a three-week-long teaching gig called "Found in France: The Artful Traveler." When we arrived at the Toulouse airport, however, I discovered to my dismay that I'd left my driver's license at home, and I was to be our designated driver. Without thinking I called Ole, asking if he'd mind going to my cottage, finding my wallet, and faxing my license to me at the car-rental place at the airport. A lot to ask of a man who hasn't yet tried to kiss you, but there was something that seemed so familiar about him, as if this request (from France!) were as natural as fishing for cats. Within forty minutes, I was behind the wheel of a Peugeot, and Sas and I were headed south. After that, Ole and I exchanged emails more frequently, almost every day. Sometimes twice.

Just before the proliferation of Wi-Fi and smartphones, I'd had to scout out the nearest Internet café to use a French keyboard (and often a deadly slow dial-up connection) to email this man who wrote sentences like he cast the fishing line. "This day in my shop has been wonderful," one email reads. "My cello bow is yielding to my urgings and coming to life. It feels like it could be a good one. The stick is strong, lively and has the lines of a pedigreed stallion. How could anyone resist it when it looks and feels so good? I love that the bows take on lives of their own. They can become the tools that unleash someone's passions for a lifetime…it's a beautiful thing."

By the time Sas and I finished teaching and arrived in Paris, I was sick with anticipation for Ole's next missive. In the course of three weeks (and from five thousand miles away), this quiet man had seduced me. Not only that, when I arrived home, he picked me up—in his parents' car—at the airport. A cooler full of groceries lay in the back seat.

Chapter 27.

∽ No Spin ∽

My neighbor Fred was delighted that I was spending more and more time with Buddy. Early on I was shy, thinking it might be an intrusion if I did too much, but Fred said I was welcome to take him to clinics and ride him whenever I wanted. "He needs the exercise, for sure. He's got a lot of energy in there," Fred said. It was clear that he wanted the best for Buddy.

One day he called and said he was taking a pack trip into the mountains for a week. He'd decided to leave Buddy behind because he only needed the two mules. "Would you mind checking on him? He doesn't like to be alone." I happily said yes and arrived at the meadow just as Fred's trailer was pulling out. Buddy was ripping around the field, whinnying as if his heart were broken. He came to a screeching stop at the fence, paused for a moment, looked down Henry Street, where the trailer had disappeared, and then wheeled toward the opposite corner and whinnied again. It was the kind of desperate call that comes deep from the belly. His whole body shook when he cried.

"Buddy!" I called from the gate. "Buddy, it's all right! They'll be back." Buddy didn't listen, though. He was too busy with his own crisis. His family was gone.

I felt terrible for Buddy. I wanted to let him know that Molly and Gracie were only gone for a week. But he didn't think that way. And then I was happily surprised when the next day Buddy only had eyes for me. He cantered right to the gate, glad for the company. I became his herd.

Ken was teaching me that there is no spin, no subtext to the messages Buddy gave. Yes, I was overjoyed that when he was happy to see me he was open and easy. And when his ears were back, he was clearly grouchy. And sometimes he was sad, just like me. Unlike humans, though, a horse has no hidden agenda. Buddy didn't lie nor did he hold a grudge. He remembered things, yes, but there wasn't a religious or moral self-righteousness about his opinions. He was what he was, even when he was a brat.

The same with misfortune. Buddy didn't complain about victimhood or how God must be punishing him or any such nonsense. In fact, I sensed he was closer to the Mysteries than most beings I knew. I began to see more clearly how he took each day and faced it head-on. Horses grieve, too, as I'd witnessed with Buddy's despair about Molly and Gracie, but it is not wrapped up with "What I should I have done to prevent this!?" or "If I'd only…"

Ken was always talking about the distinction between "I can't" and "I won't." Sometimes when a horse is afraid or traumatized, it looks like "I won't" when really it is saying "I can't." I was finding out that true horsemanship is knowing the difference.

"People often impose a false dream on a relationship with their horse," Ken told me. "They want to project their own story onto an animal who might have a very different personality from what they *want* their horse to be." So often, he said, humans want to sentimentalize their relationship with animals. Tear-jerker movies slay us with their emotional agony; it took me days to get over sad horse stories. Early on I stayed away from *Black Beauty*. Even *My Friend Flicka* took its toll. What I was coming to learn, though, is that horses are far more sophisticated than we give them credit for. Their relationship with humans is as deep as the human will go to meet them.

Buddy was showing me that adversity is not always something we can predict or control. It doesn't arise from a Big Plan, nor is it always connected to some misstep in our own actions. If I can look at events this way—as a horse does—it relieves me of magical thinking about who Buddy is, who I am. Ken warned me about making up a story around Buddy to fit some dream I had. If I projected my own stuff onto him, he said, it insulted his integrity. Of course, we humans have told stories to help ourselves make sense of our world since the beginning of time, from the Bhagavad Gita to the Bible to the Koran. I was discovering the hard way, though, that if I become too attached to a narrative, if I don't let it morph and change like a living thing, then I become a slave to—rather than liberated by—the story.

The deeper things got with Buddy, though, the more I longed for his story to be mine. And the more I invested in him, the more I conjured what-ifs: What if Fred changed his mind after the pack trip and no longer wanted me messing with his horse? What if he decided to sell Buddy to someone else? What if one day, when I arrived at Bluff Meadow, Buddy was gone?

Chapter 28.

Swimming Fast and Glorious

TWO DAYS AFTER OLE FETCHED me at the airport, he called to ask if I'd drive over and fetch him. "Can you come at 10:00 p.m.?"

"Kind of late to go out on the town, isn't it?" I'd been hoping for a romantic evening at my cottage. This man touched my body with the same attention he gave his delicate bows.

"There's a meteor shower. Bring a sweater," he said.

When I picked him up that night, I reached across the seat and poked him gently in the ribs. "But isn't the *man* supposed to pick up his date? In a *chariot*?"

"Turn left," he said, and soon we were on a dirt road that opened into a field. Ole had brought a thermos of tea and sandwiches. We parked the car, dragged out sleeping bags, and pulled on our hats and mittens, even though it was midsummer. We snuggled on the hood where the engine ticked, and we lay back on the windshield. The entire sky was filled with streams of light, and suddenly we found ourselves in the tail-end of a comet, its bits and pieces flying past, hundreds of stars a minute.

"Your poem's up there," he said. I nodded and moved closer to him. We held hands under the sleeping bags.

"By the time these stars are visible," Ole said, leaning farther back on the car windshield, "they've long been dead." An explosion of light streaked across the sky. "Ooooooh!" we said. and "Ohhhhhh!" as if they were fireworks. "Look at that one!" Swoops of light wrote themselves across the blue-black sky, as if past, present, and future were exploding in unison. When we closed our eyes, the arcs of light remained imprinted on our lids.

As the summer unfurled, Ole and I could not stay away from each other. We took breaks from our work during the day and walked the beach or read aloud to each other. At his request I'd brought a copy of Saint-Exupéry's *Wind, Sand, and Stars* from Paris. Though he knew some French, we read the English translation. One of the scenes reminded me of a Salinger story, and Ole said he'd never heard of him. I swung my leg over the arm of the sofa.

"How could anyone not know J. D. Salinger?!"

Ole turned to face me, "Here's the deal. If you are lost in the wilderness, I can get you out with a map and a compass. I don't need J. D. Salinger to do that."

On the beach a few days later, Ole named every piece of seaweed—in Latin. He'd studied biology in college. "*Nereocystis lutkean,*" he said, pointing out a thirty-foot bull kelp, wound around a rock like a giant's wild hair. He knelt down and touched some feathery, red-veined algae. "*Polyneura latissimi,*" he said, avoiding the barnacles. "You wouldn't have liked me in high school or college. I'm sure of it." He flashed me a smile. My mother would have told me to be nice to him.

Ole possessed an animal intelligence. He planted vegetable gardens and tended his cats quietly. He knew how to windsurf, he had been an oarsman for years, he said, and he casually mentioned he was taking up paragliding. I found out from a mutual friend (Ole would rather die than brag) that he'd won the county's triathlon several years before. The source of his quiet confidence was a mystery. Maybe it came from having more than one language at his service, or knowing what it is to be uprooted from your home and transported to another country. He told me he'd never forgiven his parents for taking him away at age six from the sea and mountains of Norway. Once as a five-year-old he'd sneaked out of his house and stowed away on the mailboat that sailed up the fjord-fingered coast. It took a day and a night to track him down.

He also knew how to tend the sick. His dad had been ill for several months, and, helping his mother, Ole was unafraid of bedpans, wet sheets—things I, too, was familiar with. When he talked about his bowmaking, it was like listening to a philosopher. "It all comes down to dust," he said one day, describing how one gram in a bow's weight can make or break its power. "After all, it's the magic wand for a player; it has to unlock her voice."

One morning at the end of that summer, he suggested we take a hike to the top of Mt. Townsend, one of his favorite day hikes. Dad had told me about this hike, he'd done it many times to prepare for his Olympus trip, but I hadn't been up that trail.

"Sure!" I said and joked, "Are we biking to the trailhead …?"

"Enough," he said. "Pack your backpack and pick me up in your car at my house in a half hour." We headed toward the sparkly peaks on a brilliant August morning. As we sped past the airport road, Ole reached over and touched my shoulder. "Oh, could you turn here? I have something to drop off at the airport. It will only take a second."

When I pulled up to the small air strip, he grabbed a box out of the backseat. "I'll be back in a flash. Okay? Actually, why don't you come with me?" I had to admit, this man looked great in Carhartt jeans. He didn't exactly walk; he moved like an antelope or a creature that can clear a fence. I jumped out of the car and followed him to a hangar near the gas tanks.

He slid open the huge portal, and there stood a shiny blue Cessna 150. Ole grabbed the propeller with both hands and leaned back, pulling that bird out of its nest and into the early morning sunlight. When the plane was out on the tarmac, he lifted the nozzle from the gas tank and began filling it up. He took the earphones out of the cardboard box, threw them in the pilot's seat, and opened the passenger door.

"Well? You wanted a chariot. Hop in."

I sat down on the asphalt, my mouth hanging open like the hangar door.

"It's the only time I've seen you speechless!" he said, "Get in! We'll fly over Mt. Townsend." When we lifted off the tarmac, the tiny plane bounced in the updraft. We buzzed the mountaintops and dipped toward lakes. Ole had been trained in aerobatics, he said, but he promised not to do a hammerhead.

I should have known that his fascination with Saint-Exupéry had come from a passion of his own. We swam far above our troubles with our parents, and in that little Cessna we found our own lift. Like Celia's angelfish wings, I thought, Ole and I were swimming fast and glorious.

By the following spring, the Bowmaker and I were inseparable. Nights returning from looking after Mom and Dad, I'd find a meal made and the woodstove fired up, Badge and Callie fed and happy. And every single time he came with me to see Mom, she'd smile at me, her eyebrows rising conspiratorially as she mouthed again—"Cute." All my friends liked Ole. Once when Haas and I were discussing one of the men he had a crush on, he'd said, "But Damon doesn't hold a candle to Ole. You guys are terrific together. There's no spin with him. No worries about you falling for the glitter—he's *beyond* glitter."

In April I headed to Seattle to catch a plane for a teaching gig back East. The previous night, however, I'd been stricken with a stomachache that didn't go away. "Why not stop at the doctor on the way out of town?" Ole said.

"Oh, it will probably go away," I said, hugging him goodbye, and threw my suitcase in the car.

"Just do it; you have plenty of time before your flight," he said.

I told the doctor my symptoms, and he checked me out. "Everything seems okay," he said. "But has it occurred to you that you might be pregnant?"

"I'm forty-four years old," I said, "that's hardly likely," and reluctantly told him about my previous miscarriages, skimming over the details. I did recall that the night Ole's cat Dogger had died, we'd made love to fend off the grief. I vaguely remembered that I'd been ovulating. I could tell by the pinch in my side.

"Well, let's check anyway," the doctor said, gave me a strip to check my urine, and disappeared. I sat in my gown waiting, the gray clouds outside the window. I looked at the clock. My flight was at one, and I still had a couple hours of driving ahead of me.

The doctor knocked and came in smiling. "Well. Are you ready to change your plans? Considering your history, I recommend that you not fly to Philadelphia today. Congratulations. The test is positive."

Leaving the doctor's office in a daze, I headed back home, feeling both airborne and grounded. I called Ole immediately and said, "Can you come over?"

"Now? You're home? I thought you were on your way to the airport. Did you stop at the doctor?"

When Ole moved out of his house and into my cottage, we told Rosemary and Paul our news, but not our parents. We'd contemplated moving to a bigger place, but I could not fathom leaving my safe little beach cottage, and we both hated the idea of leaving the water, so Ole said, "I'll just build our baby a hanging bed." We looked up at the tiny, two-story cathedral ceiling, the gable end with a round window framing an electric candle. We could already see the cradle swinging gently over the couch. Ole held me close as I'd never been held before. I had not one ounce of worry about his taking care of me or this glimmering beginning of a child.

All previous fears and losses were transformed by the news of this baby. The chestnut mare came to mind, as well: "There must be something better waiting for you…" Yes, I could see the whole story now—it all made sense. Our surprise baby was actually Celia's angelfish swimming fast and glorious.

Though I was dying to break our news to Mom and craved the look that would cross her face when I told her, I knew it wasn't fair. She wouldn't retain it. I'd have to tell her again and again and again. Ordinary patterns and familiar information were the most calming things for Mom, and I also didn't want to count my chicks before they were hatched. One afternoon when I took Mom on a drive, we passed a house with a slide and swing set in the front yard. Instead of pointing it out—along with the cute dog near the swing—I averted my eyes and drove on.

"Mom," I said, turning into the Point No Point Lighthouse parking lot. "What was the most wonderful surprise that happened to you in your life?" I turned off the ignition. Seagulls circled and cried, diving and swirling in the wind over the waves. Her pretty face was illuminated by the spring sun. She smiled back and said, without pausing, "Why, having you children, of course. I didn't know how much it would change my life. How much I would love you."

Chapter 29.

⤳ Cut Out the Mother ⤳

IN OLE'S NORWEGIAN FAMILY, THE first-born male names always begin with an *O*, so we agreed on his grandfather's—Olav. Every day Ole and I walked the fields and forests by the sea, keeping me fit to carry our little man of surprise. One morning, we found a pink-and-blue, hand-knit infant's bootie stuck on a thorn in the rosehips, a sign that Olav was safe with us. I untangled it from the stickers, and we brought it home. Ole stir-fried kale for the folic acid, and he insisted I rest as much as I could. Soon he was drawing plans for the cradle, which looked like a little airplane.

My body swelled. Three months into our carefully guarded secret, Ole and I knew we were nearly over the rapids. One more month and I'd be over the high-risk mark. The doctor urged me to keep calm, and Rosemary and I talked every day, giddy with the news. On Ole's and my daily walk, we watched a pair of eagles do their annual homemaking. The huge sticks and massive sculpture of their treetop aerie was visible from the field by the beach. Each spring the eagles produced one or two chicks that grew into fledglings who then flew away to start their own families.

That year, however, the eagle couple was behaving strangely. They circled nervously and rose above their nest, calling in their piercing voices. Up and up and up they circled, crying in their gyre. It was odd, we noted, that the female wasn't in the nest by now. We asked the wildlife biologist Bob about it; he knew the eagle couple intimately. Each spring and summer he stood in the field for hours with his huge telescope, counting the feedings, monitoring the eagles' activities as if they were his own family.

"This year," he told us, "The pair is too old." He held his telescope with one hand and pointed toward the nest. "They haven't been able to reproduce. Those eggs never hatched."

The birds had their ritual for grief, he said, and it was what we'd been seeing. Higher and higher they spiraled and mourned, round and round, rising on the thermals until they almost disappeared. Their calls haunted us, and we hurried home.

I carried on with my work, and one morning I drove to the Navy to teach a course called "Writing with Muscle." I left early so that I wouldn't feel rushed driving the hour and a half down the Peninsula. Just beyond the Hood Canal Bridge, a pheasant flapped out of the brush by the road. I had no time to stop. The bird hit my fender, then rolled under my car. In my rearview mirror all I could see was bright green and brown feathers. I pulled over to the shoulder. My heart fluttered and I begged for forgiveness. He was dead when I got to him, but I managed to carry him to the side of the road and lay him gently in the ferns. Cars whizzed past.

When I got to the Navy Base, I called Ole in tears. Instead of saying, "Oh, it'll be all right," he just listened. The silence on the other end was not a void, but a comfort. He just let my tears come. "The bird is not suffering now. You gave him a safe place. I'll be here when you and Olav come home. What would you like for dinner?" A warmth spread through my belly. My tilted morning was righted, and I went to the restroom to wash my face and prepare for a day of teaching.

The bloodstain on my underpants spoke to me like the grim reaper. A dreadful déjà vu. Like that day at Los Alamos, I taught sitting down all day. At lunch I drove away from the base and found a back road where a dilapidated stable stood in a field. No horses, but I pulled over and threw down a blanket. I lay on the grass, hoping against hope that I could keep Olav inside me. I didn't dare utter a prayer. Too risky. All I could think of was that poor pheasant.

A trip to the doctor the next day yet again told me the truth. Olav had left the nest.

When I called Rosemary to tell her my news, she said, "Just cry it out, Christine. Empty the bucket." After all that preparation, all the beautiful vegetables Ole had been making for me, the careful protection of my body—everything we did to make that baby safe—it still wasn't enough. What did it mean to be safe anyway? How could one protect anything in this world? Shortly after Olav disappeared, so did Ole's other cat, Lorus. I railed against a Creator that seemed like a cold Destroyer, not only of our baby, but our story. Ole and I cried together, we held each other close. We walked to the lighthouse, the wind blowing through us. One night we just sat on the beach and let the waves do the talking for us. Before we walked back to the cottage, Ole squeezed my hand and said, "It's not easy being human…"

In those days I found myself straddling the Great Divide, watching one river rush to the ocean with my mother, the other churn east to the plains with my children. Like the litany in Donald Hall's poem about his grandfather's long-dead horses, I heard the cadences of my son's names and wrote them down like a found poem: "Zeus, Joey, Olav. Zeus, Joey, Olav. Zeus, Joey, Olav."

To keep Mom from slipping away, Dad had installed special locks on the doors. But they didn't always work. Once, Mom had escaped while Lily was in the other room. Lily was frantic until she found Mom halfway down the hill walking toward the ferry.

"She keeps asking if she can go home now," Dad told me on the phone. "Even when she *is* home." In the middle of the night, Dad was now getting up and taking Mom on drives around the Peninsula in the darkness, just to assuage her desire to "go home."

"Last night I talked with her about all the homes she's had," Dad went on. "Her homes when she was a child, the farm, her homes of our early married life in Palo Alto and Seattle, the big house in Meadowdale." When he finally brought her back to Kingston, he had to convince her over and over again that "these doors are the doors to our home, Mary."

When he asked how things were going for me with Ole and the Navy gig, I could not burden my father with another sorrow. I kept the miscarriage to myself and assured him that Ole and I were great, then hung up and made a vegetable soup for dinner.

Every year in late August and early September, the Pacific Northwest salmon smell the freshwater streams of their youth, and they head back home—hundreds of miles—to spawn. Ole had taught me the double-haul cast, and his father had built me a beautiful salmon fly rod that Ole and I called the Queen Mother.

One spangled September morning when the sun was burning the mist off the sand flats, I tied one of Ole's dad's gorgeous flies on the tippet, put on my waders, and headed to the beach, determined to bring home a fish. I cast out toward the kelp beds where the salmon often hovered. I saw one jump about twenty feet from me, its scales flashing in the morning sun. I walked in so deep the waves sloshed right over the tops of my waders and cold water seeped down my trousers. Then, strangely, my reel came off my rod and sank deep down into the murky depths, the line unfurling in slow motion underwater like strands of seaweed or the tendrils of plaque attached to my mother's brain.

My sweatshirt sleeve got soaked up to my shoulders when I finally found the reel and lifted it out of the water. I attached it again and cast out toward the kelp bed and finally felt a bump on the line. Wham!! The swirls in the water and the incredible tumult of spray made my heart race, but then the line went limp.

When I arrived back at my cottage empty-handed, I checked my voicemail and found a message from Paul in Boston. "Mom has gone to the hospital," he said in an even tone. "No need for you to have known before now—the ferries would have stopped before you could have gotten there."

"Ferries?" "There?" I didn't understand, especially since I'd just spoken to Dad the previous afternoon before he and Mom were having dinner. I called Paul before listening to the rest of the message. "I guess Mom was having terrible delusions last night," he told me. "She's in the geriatric psych ward of Stevens Hospital. Dad's still there."

We thought Mom would only be at the hospital a few days, but she spent a week in the care of trained Alzheimer's doctors and nurses who administered kindness, medication, and tranquility. When I arrived to see her, I braced myself for the worst. Mom stood in the hallway looking confused, but calm. She was clutching a life-sized infant doll in pink baby clothes. The second she saw me, her face turned into the light of recognition. "You're someone I want to keep on file all day long," she laughed. I hugged her frail but familiar body.

A nurse named Elaine explained to me later that Mom had completely attached herself to that doll.

"I'm sending it with her when she leaves," Elaine whispered. According to Dr. Holmes, the staff physician, Mom could not go home. It was time, he said, for her to go to the Alzheimer's care facility, the one Paul, Rosemary, Dad, and I had finally decided on after months of searching and deliberating. My brother planned to fly out from Boston and would be there, too, when she arrived at her new digs. In negotiating the room, we had requested that Mom have a window on the Olympic Mountains side, almost the same view she had from her bedroom at home. Home. When I was a kid I was so attached to my home that, after eating the cheese and cucumber sandwich Mom had made (never a Twinkie!), I carefully folded the wax paper and banana peels or plum pits from our tree—and stowed them back in my lunchbox. I knew my crumpled napkin would be sad and lonely in the school trash with all those Hostess wrappers. I brought them home to our familiar waste bucket under the cozy kitchen sink.

Not surprisingly, Celia, too, had adopted these allegiances. I made all her Halloween costumes, and the previous year she'd requested a snail (a *red* snail to be exact). "A snail?" I'd inquired.

"So I will never have to leave home!" she said proudly. I sewed a conical tube out of the red fabric Celia had chosen at the fabric store, stuffed it with cotton candy–like batting, and coiled the tube into a fat spiral. I attached shoulder straps, so Celia could carry it like a backpack. With optic stalks waving on her headband, my niece was a magnificent snail. The final embellishment (a stroke of genius, I thought, and to this day I believe if there's a heaven I might just be admitted for this single achievement) was the five feet of Saran Wrap I attached at the last minute—a perfect slime trail. As she marched down the noisy hallway in the kindergarten parade, the small sign I'd pinned to the shell was visible to all: Home Sweet Home.

I desperately hoped that Mom, like Celia, would be happy carrying her home with her. At the end of the week, Mom was still confused, but docile about what was next, as if she were relieved of the pressure to "be normal." The staff had fallen in love with Mom and were sorry to see her go. It was decided that Dad and I would take her on the ferry back to the Peninsula and then the memory care facility not far from Kingston.

"Looking at you is looking at somebody who is easily nice to everybody," Mom said to me the last day at the hospital. I laughed, thinking it was she who was "easily nice to everybody." We wandered back to her room in the ward and sat on her bed.

"You're running around doing your work, and here I am plopped here," she continued, motioning her hand around the hospital room, "but I think I would have killed myself if I hadn't seen you coming through that door."

"Oh, Mom, me too," I said. Mom pulled her baby doll closer, straightening its little newborn hat, and we admired the doll's blue eyes. "Baby isn't real, but she's coming into who and where we are," Mom said, stroking Baby's eyelids.

It occurred to me that Mom was coming into who and where she was, too. I recalled the eloquent writing of Lawrence Weschler, who was sent in 1995 to The Hague to cover the Yugoslav War Crimes Tribunal. When he interviewed one of the judges who had heard countless hours of the most gruesome testimony a human ear can hear, Weschler asked the judge how he kept sane. "'Ah,' the judge said with a smile, 'You see, as often as possible, I make my way over to the Mauritshuis Museum, in the center of town, so as to spend a little time with the Vermeers.'" Most of us, on first glance, associate the Dutchman's paintings with a life of calm—the woman with the pitcher, the serene music lessons, the rich, yellow fabrics and lovely rooms with maps. But Weschler argues that Vermeer actually *created* tranquility. That buttery light spreading over warm interiors was done in the midst of war, plague, and Vermeer's own personal economic crisis. According to Weschler, Vermeer was literally "inventing peace."

Mom had always invented her own tranquility. When I was a senior in college, she was diagnosed with breast cancer. The night

Dad called me at my dorm to say that the biopsy had revealed cancer in both breasts, I was unable to speak on the other end of the
line. Seven male surgeons waving their scalpels had told Mom that
surgery was imminent, that it was the best way to deal with this
disease. Rather than taking their advice, however, she'd said—much
to their horror—that she'd like to think about it. Then she went
home and did some research. When she returned to the Meeting of
the Surgeons, Mom told them she'd decided against surgery. They
were outraged. They told her essentially that she was mad. "I might
be," she told them, "but I've also done a lot of reading. And praying.
I believe this is the right choice for me. Plus," she added as a throw-
away line, "I don't believe in unnecessary mutilation of the body."

Only one doctor responded to her claim on her own health. He
supported her choice to go with the new treatment (now standard
for certain kinds of breast cancer) at a Seattle cancer clinic. At
the time, only one other woman had tried what is now a common
procedure that involves a lumpectomy and high doses of intense
radiation. No surgery. Mom proceeded with this for six months.
She also championed the likes of Norman Cousins, who believed
that funny movies had sent his cancer into remission. At the same
time and on her own terms, Mom was practical about the disease.
She promptly took high doses of Vitamin C. "It couldn't hurt,"
she reasoned. She approached the months of radiation treatment,
which required a daily trip into Seattle, as an adventure. She fully
believed in the power of medicine, but also in the power of her own
decisions. In fact, when Mom was in the early stages of Alzheimer's
and the doctor had warned that hormone therapy, a new possible
antidote, was also dangerous in terms of cancer risk, she recounted
to me, "Oh, I've done breast cancer already," taking a bite of popcorn. "That seemed to turn out all right."

On the way to the ferry, September light looked like the kind
from elementary school, those days when it still seemed like

summer and a crying shame to be in class. Dad drove slowly, almost deliberately, while Mom held the baby doll in her lap. I sat in the backseat. When we got to the ferry, we decided to stay in the car during the crossing, not to cope with the usual ascent to the deck. Mom loved the ferry. Even in the rough year that had led up to this moment, every time she made the familiar crossing, she exclaimed at the light on the water, the mountains, the whales and cormorants. This afternoon we were lucky enough to be parked near the bow of the boat, and the sun slanted across our laps. We felt the breeze off the water through the open car window. I could not bear to think that this would be Mom's last ferry ride on Puget Sound. When we docked and drove off the boat, Dad turned off the main street and drove a back way to the memory care facility, so Mom wouldn't know she wasn't going home to Kingston. Mom snuggled the baby in her arms, laughed at her own charade, and quietly looked out the window. "How pretty," she said and waved her hand at the Vermeer-gold meadows.

When the three of us arrived at the memory care facility, Mom clutched her baby doll to her chest and willingly walked into the big lobby with Dad and me. Sylvia, the woman in charge, met us at the desk. We were led straightaway to Mom's clean room with the big window looking over the Olympic Mountains.

This was a brand-new facility, and there were few residents. It felt like we were rattling around in there, but the director, Gina, was full of enthusiasm. "Welcome, Mary!" she said. There was a sign on Mom's door with her name on it and flowers on her bureau. Mom smiled as if she'd arrived at another beautiful hotel with Dad. Rosemary and Paul were there, too. They had come earlier with Mom's rocking chair, a bookshelf, some pictures of Mom's father and his brothers when they were boys, and the three framed baby pictures that Dad took of us when Paul was eight, I was four, and Rosemary was a laughing infant.

"Hi, Mom!" Paul said and hugged her.

"Oh!" she said, squishing herself against Paul's huge torso.

"Isn't it beautiful?" I asked Mom with a note of nervous expectancy.

"It's as if you asked me to come and be somebody wonderful here!" Mom said and plopped down on the bed. Paul, Rosemary, and I arranged things in her room. "What a great hotel!" Mom waved her arms in a kind of dance movement—at the bed, the view of the mountains, "Ahhhhh."

Suddenly we realized that Dad had disappeared. It was never unusual for our father to slap his pockets and leave a room quickly. He always had business to do—speaking to hotel managers and making dinner reservations. And even when he didn't, he used that as an excuse to leave. He needed his space. We knew he'd gone to finish negotiations with the director, but he'd been gone an awfully long time.

"Where's Dad?" I whispered to Rosemary.

"I don't know," she said.

"I guess Dad's gone to make dinner reservations, Mom," I said out loud. Paul continued to straighten Mom's bed and show her the bathroom. We'd planned that he would stay with her for dinner. The director told us that it's best if the family divides up at this crucial transition. All of us gathering would make it seem all the emptier after we left. Since I'd made the ride with Mom and Dad on the ferry, Paul wanted to see her through her first meal.

"We think this place is just great, Mom," I said. "We all love it."

"Lyle Lovett?" she said with a twinkle in her eye. Which reminded me that we had actually brought one of her favorite Lyle Lovett tapes, and we inserted it into the boom box we'd brought for her room. He crooned about his pony in the boat, riding out across the ocean.

"Mom, let's go look at the place, shall we?"

I had a surprise for Mom. It was one of the reasons we'd chosen that facility. I led her into the hall. The room next to Mom's had a name card that read, "Lainie."

Lainie popped her head out and walked toward us, smiling.

"Mom," I held her hand, "do you know who this is?"

Mom looked confused but friendly. "Yes," she said with utter politeness, but it was clear she didn't have a clue who her next-door neighbor was.

"This is Lainie, Mom! Your college roommate!" Lainie smiled and hugged Mom. "I'm so glad to see you," Lainie giggled, as if Mom had come to her own house for a Book Club lunch, and patted her hand. Neither remembered, but they'd seen each other almost every month for half a century at their college friends' Book Club. Mom laughed, and we continued to wander around the huge common space of the Alzheimer's Unit, where the walls were painted with trees, balloons, flowers, and sky.

As we came back to Mom's room, Mom stopped. She looked at Lainie again as if seeing her for the first time, "Oh!" she said, "I think I know who you are now!" They touched each other's arms in a kind of sisterly gentleness. When we got back to Mom's room, I was nearly ecstatic with the recognition. "Mom, isn't it a hoot that Lainie's here, too?"

"Terribly hoot-like," Mom said.

When we got back to the room, Rosemary and Paul reported that after signing papers, Dad had looked stricken. All week he'd stayed at a motel near the hospital. He was emotionally and physically drained. Paul had urged him to go home and get some rest, and Dad had left without saying goodbye. I pictured him returning to his empty house, the chaos of Mom's last days there still surrounding him. Clothes scattered, dishes missing, and small things—like the lists and unearthed letters—abandoned on tabletops and strewn across the bed. Rolodex cards stuffed into her underwear drawer, the little wooden ducks she shared with Celia rattling in a box in the clothes dryer. Or the remains of her Washington State driver's license I'd found one night on her bedside table. All the vital stats were there—date of birth, address, and license number, but she had carefully clipped away her I.D. picture.

Twenty years ago, she'd sent me a photo of my Boston boyfriend and me, taken during one of her many visits East. She happened to be in the picture, too, smiling and standing next to us, evening light pouring through an open door of a concert hall. The enclosed letter had said, "Remember this wonderful night? Wasn't it *fun?* You and P. are so cute together. After you look at this, just cut out the mother."

Chapter 30.

⟶Seen and Unseen⟵

MOM'S MEMORY CARE FACILITY WAS absurdly called "Montclair Park," as if it were a mountain nature preserve or a wildlife viewing area. Celia called it "St. Mont Park," and it became our second home. We learned the code number to get in the doors (Mom's friend Lainie had figured it out already, and it had to be changed twice), and all the caregivers became our family, too: Nelcey, Donna, Ed, Nannette, Maria, Jaimie, Carmelita, Mila, Patti, and Lucy.

I began to see Mom two or three times a week if I was teaching at the nearby Navy base. She was usually asleep on her bed, her mouth wide open, her face unreadable. By six months into her residency at St. Mont Park, Mom had sunk into a kind of stupor. Most of her fellow residents, however, drifted around the facility with their own agendas. Sally in her yellow pajamas and slippers pointing at whomever she encountered, saying, "You need to leave!" Or Pegeen, a patient transferred from a state institution, who wandered into Mom's room hourly, following her thumb. It wasn't long before we were immune to such behaviors. When Pegeen drifted into Mom's room for the zillionth time (thumb straight up in the end of her outstretched arm) I'd say, "Hi Pegeen!" and continue brushing Mom's hair.

The hour's drive to St. Mont Park became a regular part of life, too. I avoided the main highway and turned left on the Big Valley Road, a stretch with old barns, big meadows, and— yes—camels. In a field not too far from the turnoff, Gobi and Cinnamon munched on grass. I knew their names because I'd stopped and asked the woman who lived next to the field. The camels' lips turned up in a smile, and they didn't seem to notice the dripping rain on their shaggy coats. I told Mom about the camels, something she would have loved in real life, but she didn't budge. She just stared off into the Land of Forgetting, far away from any here-ness. Often it was only the sound of my voice she responded to. Her eyes would flicker, and for a moment her light landed on me.

She no longer had to keep a good face for Dad, but he came every day to feed her breakfast, then sit with her in the spacious Great Room. He made friends with all the caregivers, booming across the hall to Ed or Maria. They all looked forward to his cheerful bravado and how he called everyone by name.

One afternoon Rosemary met me at St. Mont Park, and we sat with Mom, holding her hand and stroking her hair. We moved the big La-Z-Boy Maria had tucked her into so that a sunny patch from the clerestory windows could touch her face. I read aloud the Nursery School report cards Paul had emailed me from Boston that morning. His twins, Margie and Libby, "love to dance," I read, and they were doing well "sharing" and "cleaning up." Then Mom fell asleep, and Rosemary and I hurried to meet our appointment with her doctor. Dad had had a long meeting with him that week and wanted us "to hear what he has to say about Mom's future."

Dr. D., who specialized in gerontology, was an hour and a half late to our appointment. We were just about ready to leave when he hurried in, a dark-skinned, middle-aged man. His intelligent eyes met ours with an immediate apology.

"I am so sorry I'm late. There are not enough hours in the day." He sat down, opened Mom's chart, and looked directly at us. He also opened both hands, palms up. "Please. Tell me your questions."

Soon Rosemary and I realized we were in the presence of someone who had thoughtfully worked through what he called "End-of-Life Issues." He cut to the chase.

"Alzheimer's patients are never going to get better. Ever," he said.

"Why is Mom so sleepy all the time?" I asked, trying to avoid the thought of Mom not ever getting better.

"It's not the drugs she's taking for anxieties or seizures," he said, "but your mother is in—the final stages of this disease." He paused. "It's not an attractive word, but your mother is in a 'vegetative stage.' She has lost almost everything now. The last thing that will go is knowing her own name. That is really the most primary thing we learn. Our name." He sat back in his chair and laid the clipboard on his lap.

Rosemary and I pictured Mom smiling every time Maria, her favorite caregiver, uttered "Mary."

Then Dr. D. gently brought up a term we were not familiar with: "Code Status." It outlined how much medical intervention would be administered should Mom have an infection or the flu.

"It's important that families clarify the Code Status," he said, "so your mother will be treated with palliative care." The only intervention, he told us, would be for pain or dry lips.

"Pretty soon she will stop eating and drinking," Dr. D. explained. "That is when I recommend we allow her to…ah…"

"Press on?" I said.

"Um, yes. Press on."

Rosemary and I were oddly relieved by his clarity, which seemed to dovetail with his empathy. We knew Mom would approve wholeheartedly, and it seemed like we'd been saying goodbye to Mom for so long—nearly five years—that Death was fashioning himself as a welcome guest.

Dr. D. also mentioned that we, as Mom's daughters (and our brother, too), probably worried about our own health when it came to dementia. In unison Rosemary and I nearly shouted, "Yes!" then laughed nervously. There had yet to be any definitive research that proved there was a genetic link, but it hovered in the news and in the back of our minds. There'd been a recent report that beer might have something to do with Alzheimer's, and we'd been feeling fated to get it. How many brews had we drunk in our adult life? Besides, who wanted to give up beer? It seemed one of the few "palliative care" measures we ourselves could enjoy in the face of life's Russian Roulette of Disease and Destruction.

"Well," he laughed. "Sometimes the people who tend to drink too much beer are more likely to get dementia anyway. I wouldn't worry. But there are things one can do to fend it off."

Dr. D. shifted in his chair. "There's such a thing as 'collateral brain,'" he said. "That means that there are many paths of learning our brain can take. People say to me, 'Why is it that a circuit judge has Alzheimer's? She used her brain her whole life!' And that is indeed a good question." Dr. D. picked up his pencil and tapped it on the clipboard.

"But that judge may have been using only the *analytical* side of her brain. Artists, for example, have less of a chance of developing dementia for that very reason. Musicians, too. They use many different pathways of the brain. It's called 'recruitment.'"

I nearly leapt up off my chair and kissed Dr. D's face.

There have been other moments like this—in college, for example—when I had one-to-one conferences with my European Intellectual History professor. We'd be discussing my paper about Camus and the existential imperative of free will when, in the quiet of his oak-filled office, I'd suddenly entertain the possibility of shattering the rarefied air. In my thrill about our conversation and the intoxicating connection of new ideas, I was afraid I would (without warning) leap onto Professor Duvall's desk, kick the neatly stacked papers in all directions, and sing at the top of my lungs. As I considered this little scenario, my heart would race, and I could no longer concentrate on *The Plague* or anything but preventing what seemed like inevitable pandemonium.

"And also," Dr. D. cleared his throat as if sensing my impulse, "Recruitment happens in people who do crossword puzzles." During Mom's illness Rosemary had taken up the *New York Times* crossword with a kind of evangelical fervor. She was already a master of the Saturday puzzle. Rosemary's arms rose, and I was sure that she, too, was about to throw herself, full-bodied, into this unsuspecting gerontologist.

Luckily, Dr. D. steered the discussion back to Mom's care, and he suggested we get in touch with hospice.

"But Mom isn't dying *now*," I said. "And hospice needs a six-months-to-live diagnosis from the doctor. Can we predict that?" It was beginning to sound grim again.

"No, but if you open the case, and if she doesn't die in six months, you can open the case again and continue. Hospice care might also assume some of the costly duties at the memory care unit, as well." In addition, he said, they would provide some counseling that could help us in the "next stage."

After we left Dr. D., Rosemary, and I met Dad for dinner and discussed the things he had learned the previous week.

"Code status, Dad." I said, "It sounds like the Homeland Security paint box: Code Yellow, Code Orange…" Dad smiled and agreed. But, like the days shortly after 9/11, it was hard to predict when the siege would come.

The three of us sat on the sunny deck of Main Street Ale House drinking a glass of white wine. Dad looked terribly tired, sleepy-dirt lodged in the corners of his eyes.

"This is not getting better," he admitted. "I'm finding it really hard to go every morning and feed Mom breakfast. It's so sad," he dusted the bread crumbs off his own lap, "wiping her mouth." It seemed impossible that just a year or so before he'd almost made it to the top of Mt. Olympus. Now he was having trouble breathing when he walked up the hill from the ferry.

Rosemary and I encouraged him to take a break from meals at St. Mont Park for a while, to go when Mom was asleep. He agreed, although his sense of love and duty, especially at mealtimes, had given his life structure within Mom's absence at home. He admitted to being relieved he was no longer Mom's caregiver, but he suffered the loneliness of a widower—without the resolution of his spouse's death.

"Some of my best visits with Mom have been when she's asleep," Rosemary said. I agreed. I loved sitting next to her bed and holding her hand while I looked at the mountains, listening to her breathe. But breathing was to end soon, according to Dr. D. And—though the three of us were facing Mom's decline more honestly—we all knew that when she finally did "press on" there would be another Big Valley Road to navigate. No getting around it. And I was pretty sure Gobi and Cinnamon wouldn't be there, either.

I did, however, have a gut feeling that we were being looked after somehow, in a mysterious way we couldn't articulate. Words from the *Book of Common Prayer* came to mind, from the many years I'd heard and said the Nicene Creed: "We believe in one God…maker of heaven and earth, of all that is, seen and unseen."

When I went to see Mom later that week, the sun slanted through the blinds over her bed, creating furrows of light across her body. Her face was again lax with sleep, but when I touched my hand to her face and quietly said, "Mom," her eyes flickered and she focused. When she saw me, she smiled and said, "Ohhhhhhhhh." I pressed the handheld bed control, and the engine hummed while the upper part of her body rose gracefully.

"I wish you were always here," she laughed.

I sat on the edge of the bed. "But Mom, I am. I'm always in your heart."

"Yes, but then I have to think about it to put it in there." We laughed again. I absorbed the truth of that, how difficult the arrangement of the world was for her. Eternal in a way. Now. All the time. For her to think of something outside of "now" was less and less possible. Maybe that wasn't such a bad thing. She didn't seem agitated or sad anymore, just accepting of her fate.

I picked up the plastic horse that Rosemary had bought her. Mom had fixated on one of Celia's horses, the kind I never liked as a kid, the ones girls put on their knickknack shelves. Mom had carried Celia's horse around so much that Rosemary just bought her one.

"Look at this, Mom," I lifted the horse from his paper stable on her dresser.

"Ohhhhhhhhhhhhh," she replied, reaching for the horse, holding it on its side, and looking at it with wonder. Then she took her index finger and started rubbing the horse's dished face. Back and forth, back and forth. The same way we'd reveled in the perfect shape of Lightfoot's Arabian head.

"I like to do this," Mom smiled. "You could just put him in a buttonhole, couldn't you?"

Yes, I thought, imagining myself threading through that buttonhole and emerging into bright light. Maybe I'd find Lightfoot as well as Mom. She was hinting at something she seemed to know, even in her altered state—or maybe because of it: we are not confined to the physical world, that what and who we love can move anywhere, even through the narrow slit of a buttonhole.

Chapter 31.

⟿ *Passport* ⟿

AT SEVENTY-SIX, MY FATHER WAS still a strong man. And yet he was having trouble with night sweats and strange flu-like symptoms. It was not like my father to be sick. He was always the rock of the family. The year my father turned seventy, I'd written him a poem that compared him to the white, snowy peaks he'd scaled and how his journeys were part of "my own map in the making." But I was wrong.

It was my mother who was my map. My father was actually the compass. Charts and maps rely on the use of language and nuance; naming things helps us to get our bearings. Words attach themselves to places like "Mt. Olympus"; "Edmonds, Washington"; "South Fork of the Stillaguamish River." Unlike the map, the compass is never limited to a particular geography or a page. It's not even informed by elevation or terrain. It is portable, nomadic, and keeps its own bearings. Even in the darkest hour, when you cannot see to read, that little arrow points to the truth. My father's unerring will and sense of direction was like that compass. There is no arguing with North.

In his midsixties, he unfolded a United States road atlas, took out a ruler, and drew a straight line from Cape Flattery, Washington, to Key West, Florida. "It's downhill all the way!" he boomed. Then he'd driven that line—from the westernmost point in the continental United States to its eastern conclusion. Alone.

"I made a rule: No going beyond fifty miles either side of that line," my father told us. This self-imposed line required that he use many small roads, sometimes even logging roads. He recorded notes on a handheld recorder, documenting his thoughts and conversations with people along the way. At the halfway point in Nebraska, he found a chunk of cottonwood and buried it where he could find it again.

"I'll pick it up when I drive the other way," he said. "In a few years, I'll complete a X across the country—from Maine to California! I'm calling it 'America on the Diagonal.'"

His trips were always a way to sort out his life and his own geography. The small towns and bars, the river boatmen, the drive-in movies. "America on the Diagonal" was a theme, really, and he took pleasure in having been to those places, just as exotic as the Far East had been for him, or to Bulgaria and the Grand Cayman Islands. I think my father loved *saying* he'd been to these places. In his office he always had a map of the world with thumbtacks marking all corners of the globe where he had been.

A year after Mom was admitted to St. Mont Park, my father embarked on another diagonal journey, one for which he had no map or compass. After a number of tests for his night sweats, unusual fatigue, and difficulty breathing, he was finally diagnosed with chronic lymphocytic leukemia, CLL. I never doubted he could lick it. Even at seventy-five, his immense power—six foot four and a will of iron—resembled the mountains he'd climbed. Plus, the doctor said it was a kind of leukemia that people lived with. After what we'd been through with Mom, this was good news.

Dad and I sat in the oncologist's office and discussed treatment. A laconic man in his early fifties, the doctor shuffled papers impatiently and told us that with chemotherapy the odds for a "quality of life" were quite high. He offered us a video to prove it. Dad and

I stuffed ourselves into the viewing booth while the falsely cheerful narrators in "Living with CLL" gave advice on how to handle things like "family activities" and "outcomes."

After the film and back at the doctor's office, Dad said, "Several of my friends have really suffered with chemotherapy. I've seen them in worse shape from the medicine than from the cancer. What would happen if I didn't do the treatment?"

The doctor looked at my father as if he'd just spit up a hairball. "You would die," he said. "My job is to keep you alive; this is the only smart choice."

"But has anyone actually chosen *not* to take this course?" My father folded his hands in his lap. The doctor paused in horror, then shook his head. "No," he said, closing dad's file. He assured my father that treatment would make his life better, not worse, and ushered us out the door.

As Dad began the chemo treatment, my siblings and I had utter confidence in his staying power. We were used to Mom needing our attention, not the "Monolith," as Mom called him. When he contracted an infection, and had to be hospitalized, even then it was hard to picture this force of nature suppressed. But when I arrived at his bedside, he lay flat on the bed, the flimsy bedclothes barely covering his commanding frame.

My father fumbled with the straw in his water glass and groaned when he was asked by a nurse to turn over. With my mother fading into the Land of Forgetting and my father down with this infection, I struggled to keep my bearings. Intellectually, we all know that our parents will falter, age, and die, but even my mother's illness did not prepare me for Dad's sudden collapse. I sat in the chair close to his bed and looked out the window at sheets of rain and waited for Paul to arrive from Boston.

The infection soon turned into pneumonia, and Dad's condition floundered. High fever made him punchy, and he claimed to see people we didn't see. He gasped with pain every time he tried to roll over. Rosemary had strung up twinkly lights in the gloomy room and made a photo collage of palm trees, sunny beaches, and cool drinks on a tray. But Dad claimed that the man in one picture was threatening him, and he was "afraid of what might happen to the children." Paul removed the poster.

The sound of saws and banging on the hospital floor below shook the room as construction workers renovated the ICU. The crash of crumbling concrete accompanied the flurry of nurses who came and went with potions and notions. As Paul, Rosemary, and I discussed our father's precarious state, our thoughts were drowned by jackhammers. At one point I grabbed a nurse and asked if that noise could stop. "We don't have any control over it!" she said. And when I inquired if my father's pain and discomfort were normal in this kind of treatment, she tipped her head vaguely, "I don't know." Dad's oncologist was out of town.

"This is exactly what I did *not* want to happen," my father uttered from his damp, rumpled sheets. He waved his hand at the tray of pale food made even less appealing under the fluorescent lights. "Do I want *this* to be my life?" We left him to sleep, and we all three departed —I alone, and Paul to stay with Rosemary for the night. Riding the ferry boat across the Sound, I felt a surge of tides larger than the sea.

The next morning, my brother called and said, "You have to come right away; Dad says he has something important to tell us. He won't tell Rosemary and me until you are here." I leapt into my car and drove the three hours back to Seattle, a new sense of hope in my heart: Dad is better! He's going to leave the hospital! When I arrived my father was radiant, sitting up in bed and smiling, his powerful forearms taut. His hands gripped the handrail. Dad shooed the nurses out and swung his legs over the edge of the bed so he could sit up and command the room. We were mute with shock. Like Lazarus, our father appeared to have risen from the dead.

His lips were chapped, but they formed the words with certitude.

"I've made a decision," he said. We leaned forward, expecting the inevitable Peter Hemp Problem-Perceived-Problem-Solved solution.

"I had an epiphany in the night," he closed his eyes. "I was awake and sick of the noise going on below and the madness of this hospital. But then I heard singing…" We had a brief question whether Dad had been hallucinating. But his story had none of the feverishness of the previous night; he was as cogent as if he were at the head of the dinner table reporting his day to Mom.

"I looked up," my father raised his hand. "And the night nurse—an African American woman named Christy (almost your name, Christine!)—she was singing a spiritual as she moved around my room…It was absolutely stunning." Dad paused and took a breath. "I said to her, 'Could you sing that louder?' She told me she'd love to and closed the door quietly. Suddenly everything stopped." Dad looked up at the ceiling.

"She opened her throat and 'Amazing Grace' filled the room. It was so beautiful…" My father stretched his arms out to his sides, his hospital gown draping like a Roman soldier's tunic off his strong shoulder. His eyes glowed not only with tears, but with a clarity we had not seen in months.

"Right then," he pushed away the bed sheet from his thigh, "in the middle of her melody, I felt as if I were being freed; a huge weight was lifted off of me." He took another long breath. "I realized that I don't have to do this! I don't have to have chemo anymore. I don't have to do this awful hospital…" We all flinched as a jackhammer again vibrated up through the floor.

A nurse burst into the room. "Mr. Hemp! It's time for your shot!" My father turned to her politely, "I'm not taking any more medicine. I am having a family meeting. Please let us be alone, if you will."

"But this is the right temperature and time for…" My father held up his large hand, palm toward the nurse. "I said that was it.

Thank you. Please leave us alone now." The nurse backed out the door, muttering.

My father conveyed such a presence that we all remained quiet. I could not gather any words, but the air in the room felt suddenly fresh. And, even though Dad was delivering frightening news, the way he framed it made it sound like a victory. In those few, short minutes, my father had left the realm of victim and had pulled our family back to a familiar equilibrium. Against the advice of protesting nurses and without even telling his oncologist, my father was unplugging himself from the bureaucracy of the medical system, demanding that he be released not only from the lunacy of hospital life, but from life as we know it.

"Are you afraid to die?" I asked him later. He shook his head, "Nooooo," as if waving off a trip to the dentist. "I sent three children to college, I did some great ad campaigns, I climbed quite a few mountains and had a wonderful marriage and family. I think I've done everything I've wanted to do in this life."

Dad had always steered clear of being a Captain Bring-Down. And his resolve created a new strength in me, as if I were part of a winning plan, one in which there were no forces controlling us. No jackhammers, no unfriendly nurses, nor doctors talking down to us.

That afternoon, before we transported Dad to hospice, another oncologist, a slim, sharp woman in her early forties, came in and reported what she'd heard from the nurse, that Mr. Hemp was leaving the hospital without the approval of his doctor. "Sir, I see that your doc is out of town, and I'm filling in while he's gone. Is it true that you no longer wish to take the medication? Antibiotics or chemotherapy?"

"That's right," Dad said.

"But, Mr. Hemp, do you realize what this means?"

"My daughter Rosemary has already arranged for hospice." My father patted the mattress.

"But you can't just leave, especially without your physician's approval."

"I most certainly can," my father said, the tubes dangling free of his arms. "I am leaving today. But tell me, Dr.—what did you say your name was?"

She offered her name and said, readjusting her tone, "I am here to answer your questions."

"What will happen to me? How will it end?"

"Well," she took a short breath and relaxed her shoulders, obviously framing a sentence she had not had to do before, "since you have pneumonia, your lungs will slowly fill with liquid. It will become harder and harder to breathe. And finally, you will not be able to draw your own oxygen." My father nodded, absorbing these facts.

"Thank you so much, Dr. S.—I appreciate your honesty. I will get ready to go now."

"You must have been president of your company, Mr. Hemp." She shook her head. "I've never been forced to let a patient take this route before. Ever. It's a pleasure to meet you." She reached out her hand, and my father held it tight.

Before we left the room, Dad recited a poem, one I didn't know, and neither did Paul or Rosemary (who, unlike me, were both English majors).

"Hey!" Dad said, "Who wrote this? Just guess. And it's *not* John Keats—"

> If I were to die tomorrow night
> And I thought there were things I never might
> Be able to do again.
>
> I'd take myself down to the sea
> Where the wind and the waves crash endlessly
> And seagulls laugh at men.

"Dad," I said, "that's terrific. When did you memorize that? Who wrote it?"

"Me! Circa 1947." He lay back down in bed and closed his eyes. "Okay, I need to rest now."

The Hospice Center—which my father called "The Hyatt Regency"—was located just a couple of miles from Rosemary's, outside of Seattle. It was filled with caregivers who offered milkshakes and massaged my father's hands. The mood in the place struck me as miraculous, even though it was a house of death. "A lot different from that hospital!" Dad announced from his bed brimming with crisp pillows and comforters. Dad even decided we should have a party. Rosemary, Freddie, Celia, Paul, Ole, and I made pasta in the communal kitchen. We ate in Dad's room and watched the light fade on the naked birch trees out the window while J. S. Bach played on the CD. Dad loved Bach, but on that dark January afternoon, the familiar ordered melodies marched toward a somber fugue. Rosemary had bought Dad a fleece vest so that he could stay warm in bed, and we tried to keep up the cheer. What struck me, however, was how the warmth in that building burned stronger than the fire in the lobby fireplace. All along the corridors in hushed rooms, family and friends sat quietly with those they loved, savoring each day, each hour, each minute.

When I was a teenager, in summer I rode Lightfoot on the beach most every day. At low tide we'd gallop miles down the sandbar, which looked as if it stretched all the way to Whidbey Island. One morning I rode bareback as the mist rose off the tide flats. No one was around, and as I gave Lightfoot more rein, his Arabian gait kicked in—that floating gallop I saw the first day I'd set eyes on him. That gallop is more about lungs than legs. We flew down the shimmering sand, reveling in our partnership, knowing each other's every movement. A flick of an ear, a slight touch with my bare foot.

When we slowed down to an easy canter, the fog lifted and the summer sun burned through. I let him cool at a walk, and then I guided him toward the water. A neighbor girl's horse had drowned in that bay because she'd swum him in a martingale, a piece of tack used to keep a horse's head from lifting too high. That event had terrified me, even though I hadn't witnessed it, and I was always careful to trust Lightfoot's own instincts in the swells.

The sea rushed up over my knees and Lightfoot began to groan. I loosened the reins and his nose dabbed the water's surface. Waves moved past us and suddenly his feet left the shore and he lurched up and forward like a merry-go-round horse. Then I completely loosened the reins, holding tight to his mane so I wouldn't get washed off his back. His nostrils flared, and the full intake of his breath expanded his ribs underneath me. Lightfoot groaned again, and—with a surge of his legs in the dark water below—seaweed, tail, and mane all rushed and swirled in a churning mass of horse and water. No longer was I a girl on a horse's back. I was riding life itself.

As my father plunged into dying, his lungs began to fill; the sound of his labored breathing infused the room with a tidal rhythm.

In my family we always went as a group to the airport to pick up whoever was coming home from Boston, London, or Lagos. But we'd made a pact years before not to belabor farewells, so we'd send the departing traveler to the airport by shuttle. "No sad goodbyes!" my father would boom from the park-n-ride lot.

This time was different. We'd see Dad to the gate.

Dad also wanted to speak to Ole privately. He told him that he wanted to contribute some money toward purchasing our beach property, a lot we'd found right next to Ole's old rental house. Dad also said how relieved and happy he was that Ole and I were together. When Ole emerged from the room, his eyes were shining.

"Dad, is it hard having us all here?" I asked when we were alone. The martini he'd asked for sat on the dinner tray untouched, drops of condensation sliding down the glass.

"Are you kidding?!!" Dad said. "This is the best three days of dying I've ever had!"

Dying, like climbing a mountain, involves endurance and a lot of emotional strength. It is an act of courage. Unlike climbing a mountain, however, where one can roughly gauge the time it will take, dying is a mystery. Mom, whom we expected to press on ages ago, was still with us, and here was our rock of a father slapping his pockets and leaving the planet.

When we were finished with dinner, I offered to stay the night with Dad. There was a fold-out sofa in the room, and I had brought my laptop, a copy of Tennyson's "Crossing the Bar," and my pillow. I tried to read, but my eyes kept flitting over to check on my father, whose breath was labored and deep, sometimes punctuated by a guttural groan. Often he'd reach up above his head for something I could not see. He took off all his clothes and kicked the sheets off his naked body. The night nurse told me when people are dying, they don't want to be encumbered; they want to exit this world cleanly, with nothing holding them back. My father's naked body looked as strong as ever, and I could still hardly believe he was sick. No withering away for him. Near dawn, when he returned briefly to the conscious plane, Dad thanked me for looking after him and asked how I learned how to do it.

"What? To do what, Dad?"

"Taking such good care of me. Where did you learn that?"

"Well, I learned it from you, Dad. You always took such good care of me."

"I always will," he said.

The tides of that night moved through altered time and space. When my father woke again, he said, "Check, please!" and waved his hand toward an invisible waiter. I gave him the nearest thing I could find, one of many cards sent from close friends who were dumbfounded that Peter Hemp was leaving the party. I found a pen and Dad scribbled a bit on the card and then passed it to me, exhausted. "Will you sign it, Christine?" I did as he asked. The hospice nurse came in with a cool washcloth for my father's forehead, and he sank back into the huge business of getting himself to the other side. I trusted him. My father knew how to travel.

In the crepuscular early-morning hours, I cooled my father's forehead and held his hands. I found myself breathing deeply with him, the exhale as powerful as that life-giving intake of breath. It made me keenly aware—and less afraid—that I, too, would stop breathing someday. If my father can do this, I thought, so can I. His breath came heavier, the intake deep, loud, and labored like a horse swimming in the sea. He was willing himself to cross that bar. Such resolve and stamina transcended any mountain ascent. I could almost hear the wind around the pinnacles.

Not long before dawn, my father spoke of airplanes, flight plans, and at one point he asked me if he had his passport.

"Yes, Dad," I said gently. "You have it. No problem." I smoothed the coverlet over his chest.

"But what about you?" His voice carried the same urgency of the one in charge of travel plans. "How will you get there?"

"Don't worry, Dad," I reassured him, stroking his solid forearm, "I have my passport, too. I'll be there. I'll just be on a later flight."

PART III:
LAND OF LIVING

Chapter 32.

Memory and Desire

THE FIRST TIME I SAW Buddy I nearly spilled my coffee. Just a few months after losing Olav, Ole and I were having breakfast and reading the paper. A July breeze whispered through the open deck door of the cottage. I looked up from the newspaper to see, framed by the window, a little spitfire Arabian horse prancing down the road lickety-split. The rider, our neighbor Fred, sat calmly on a swirl of white mane and tail. I jumped up and raced out to the deck just as the horse disappeared around the corner toward the beach. I wondered if it was an apparition, my childhood friend returning to greet me. Involuntary words formed on my lips: "Glory be to God for dappled things." My pulse still quickened every time I saw a horse that even remotely resembled Lightfoot.

In my teenage years, Lightfoot had been my passport to adventure. At school I counted the minutes to when I'd finally get to step off that school bus, dash home to get changed, fetch my horse, and ride as far as I could go—along the beach, or into the woods, riding the trails till dark.

I marvel now at the trust between Lightfoot and me. I sat on him while he ate supper in the barn at night. I rode him around the meadow without a halter or bridle, guiding him only with my legs. I could even race up from behind and vault over his hindquarters to land on his back. I believe there is an innate intelligence in children, one that instinctively knows about union with an animal, the wholeness of things. We seem to unlearn that as we get older.

When high school rolled around, I was still involved in 4-H and showed Lightfoot at the fair, but I was also a class officer and sang in the swing choir, performing at venues as far away as Portland and Spokane.

"Don't forget your horse," Mom said, as I rushed out to meet friends.

"Oh, don't worry," I said, determined not to admit that I was growing up. Confused by my conflicting allegiances, I blocked out my fear that Lightfoot was being left behind, that somehow I was becoming someone else, someone more worldly than the twelve-year-old who had fallen for a horse in a mountain meadow.

As my senior year unfolded, I was accepted early decision at a small college in Oregon. Originally, we thought I'd attend Washington State University and learn about equine medicine or horse training, but I ended up applying to a liberal arts college like my brother and parents, so taking Lightfoot with me to college became less and less a possibility.

One day Mom gently suggested that we might want to find a good new home for Lightfoot. "WHAT?!" I said, "Can't he just stay here?!"

"Lightfoot is smart and young and still full of promise," Mom said. "Don't you want him to continue living his life?" The words stung. I left the house, saddled up my horse, and rode him on the beach, talking it out with him about what was the next best step. I was *not* going to be one of those girls who sold her horse when she went off to college.

There were days I was so busy with school I couldn't get to Lightfoot until late. I'd feel guilty, and, when I was guilty and sad, I closed my heart, ashamed that I'd neglected him—not in terms of feeding or care, but emotionally. Like any teenager, I learned to close my heart to the things that might hurt me, like the terrible crush I had on my classmate Dean Fredrickson.

There was something else, too. I found myself getting impatient with Lightfoot and expected things of him that I didn't know myself. One day I went to a vacant lot to lunge him with a long rope, something I'd done from time to time. I sent him out to the end of the line while I stood in the center of the circle. He trotted around, and then I asked him to canter. When he refused I smacked him with the end of the rope and he reared, pawing the air. I was just as shocked at myself as I was at his response. He was grouchy. And, like a girlfriend who knows she has to break up, I'd pushed him too hard, his response justifying my need to pull away.

Mom finally said, "Christine, I think it's time..."

Mom found a woman who immediately adored Lightfoot, and she planned to keep him at a fancy stable in Everett and train him as a jumper. Mom said the lady was gentle and kind, ecstatic to have such a handsome, intelligent animal. But to this day I cannot remember meeting her or even watching that trailer leave with my beloved horse. I blocked it out. I slathered my heart with wax and planned for my Big Life ahead.

The sight of Buddy's swishy white tail disappearing around the corner to the beach set off an unexpected longing; the moment was visceral. Though I'd ridden several horses since Lightfoot—a leggy jumper when I'd lived in England and a black quarter horse in Riojos—no horse had stayed in my cells as Lightfoot did. A dozen questions came into my head. Why hadn't I seen this horse in the neighborhood before? Where did he live? Didn't my neighbor Fred have only mules? And why did I have to agitate old memories? Why couldn't my past horse-life just stay stuck in a nice, well-framed scrapbook? But such is the nature of desire.

Later, when I ran into Fred at the mailbox, I asked about the horse. He told me he'd bought him from a woman in town, someone who'd rescued the gelding and a pony from an exotic animal farm. I pictured that horse trotting around with camels and flamingos. Fred said he kept him at a meadow up the bluff with his mules. I was relieved; I wouldn't be tantalized. In fact, when I came to my senses, I locked that desire in a safe. Somewhere between no and no.

Chapter 33.

Renaissance

I STOOD OUTSIDE MOM'S DOOR at St. Mont Park with Mom's favorite caregiver, Maria. "I can't believe Peter is gone," she whispered. "No one even knew Mr. Hemp was ill. He never told us a thing." Her soft, dark Peruvian eyes filled with tears. She said that Dad had given them all an extra hug the last day he'd seen them, and he'd lingered with Mom longer than usual. Of course, when he was first admitted to the hospital and then to hospice, we'd called St. Mont Park to let them know the turn of events. Maria had offered to bring Mom across Puget Sound so she could see Dad one last time, but he would have nothing of it. "That would be too hard on her," he'd said. End of story.

"He wanted me to stay longer, too," Maria told me, about the last day she'd seen him. "He asked me not to go on my break, something he'd never done before. I'm so glad I stayed with him and Mary that day. He must have known something." Maria shook her head. "But not only Peter knew," Maria turned her head toward Mom's open door. "Mary knew, too."

Maria told me that the evening of Dad's death, she'd heard Mom chatting alone in her bed. "I wondered who could be in there at that hour," Maria went on. "Mary hadn't spoken for such a long,

long time. Except for little words here and there. You know. She has been mostly sleeping for nearly a year now."

Maria had stepped into the room and found Mom in a long conversation with someone, very animated in her distinct and melodic gibberish.

"Mary?" Maria said, looking around the room. "Who are you talking to?"

Mom looked up and, in a voice as clear as water, said, "Peter."

When I was ten, my father taught me how to draw in three dimensions. He told me that in the Renaissance, a time of great blossoming in art, philosophy, and discovery, European painters had learned how to ground objects in three-dimensional space, so that trees did not float, and the horse remained firmly planted on the road. It was called perspective, he said. He showed me how easy it was, first drawing two vertical parallel lines. Then, in contrast, he drew those same lines as a two-sided triangle where the lines meet in what he called the vanishing point. He commandeered the black grease pencil, slashing crosspieces onto the upside-down V.

"See?" he said, the penciled ties magically turning a triangle into a railroad track disappearing on the horizon.

And here was Maria telling me that Dad—and now Mom—had stretched even further our perception of three dimensions. Though Dad was a man deeply grounded in the physical world, during his dying he'd led me right to the edge of the next one.

Celia had her own take on this. Not long after her grandfather's death, she told me, "We humans haven't really explored very far from our Earth…really. The moon is our coastline." Dad's death changed the geography of our family, but his departure seemed to expand rather than shrink mom's coastline. Like a sixteenth-century explorer, she arose to a New World. Where before she was mute, she began to talk. Where before she slept, she came into a new flowering, her own Renaissance. Maria and the other caregivers reported that Mom was smiling again, shedding her death mask for a sunny face and a laugh when anyone said her name.

One day when I couldn't visit, I called, and Janice, one of Mom's morning caregivers, answered the line. "In all my years as a nurse, Christine, I've never seen someone with dementia change for the better."

I switched the phone to my other ear, and Janice proceeded to tell me that Mom was really turning around. "Yes. I mean—it's unexplainable," she said. "Sometimes I guess the senses just come back toward the end of life." I had noticed it, too, but Janice told me something I did not know. She told me that the day before Mom was actually reading. "She was looking at *Reader's Digest* in the main room with Lainie. They were reading magazines together! I just can't figure it out!"

I asked Janice about Mom's new desire to get out of bed. In the preceeding months, she couldn't go anywhere but in a wheelchair. But now, according to the caregivers, she insisted on walking.

"Peter must be right there encouraging her," Janice said. "She's standing tall."

Janice was stretching it a bit. Mom couldn't walk entirely without help. Yet just weeks before, she'd been totally numb to the world, unable even to help the staff move her from her bed to the wheelchair to go to dinner.

"I've spent so much time around death and dying and old people—I mean, what is old age anyway? What do we know? What does it do to us? We haven't a clue, really." A mutual silence on the line briefly reflected our wonder. "Your mother is so beautiful," Janice said before we hung up. "We just love her. Hey, she might go tomorrow, but you should know that today she is really happy."

After divvying up our parents' library (I gladly claimed all the Will James books), Paul, Rosemary and I made a stack of books that Mom might like. Now that she was "reading" again, I hauled in a big box—met by the stares of the Alzheimer's residents—toward Mom's tiny room. From outside her door I could see she was resting on her bed, chatting with someone I could not see. No one was there, but she was laughing and carrying on. She stopped, as if waiting for an answer, then continued agreeing and nodding her head.

"Hi, Mom!" I said, coming in and dumping the load of books.

"Ohhhhhhhhhhhh," she said, her face lighting up when she saw me. I helped her to sit up, and we looked at *The History of the Arabian Horse* and a tattered paperback of *The Collected Poems of Robert Frost*, which radiated a dog-pound exuberance, as if the books themselves were glad to be saved from the used book store.

"Ooooooooooooooooooooo. Nice!" Mom said.

I read her a few lines from one of her Frost favorites:

I'm going out to clean the pasture spring;
I'll only stop to rake the leaves away.

Mom smiled, nodding with Frost's cadences.

(And wait to watch the water clear, I may):
I sha'n't be gone long. —You come, too.

Frost's invitation had been a familiar one to all of us kids. Mom's lit-up face gave me hope that she was still here, that she was coming, too.

"You're doing okay, aren't you, Mom?" I said.

"Oh, yes…"

"Have you been talking to Daddy?"

Mom paused only a split second. "Oh, of course I have…"

"He's pretty happy now?" I ventured into unknown pastures. She reached over and gently touched the poem on the page. "Seems to be…"

One afternoon I walked her into the Great Room to sit in the sun. She was wearing a pink sweater—who knows whose it was. The residents either stole or wore other people's clothes anyway, and clean laundry was more important than the labels Rosemary and I had so carefully sewn into Mom's outfits.

Next to Mom sat Betty, who was fondling Mom's blue-eyed Baby, the very one Mom had brought from the hospital. She slept with that doll every night, but somehow Betty had wrangled it. A proprietary urge gushed through me, and I spied another doll on the floor.

"See?" I held the new doll up to Betty. "Nice baby." I tried to wrest Mom's precious infant from Betty's claws, but she wasn't fooled. She held tighter.

Mom watched with fascination as I finally unfolded Betty's fingers one by one from Baby's head. "This is Mary's baby," I said, finally jerking the doll free and poking the other baby into Betty's open hands. "This is Mary's baby," I said again, as if to convince myself that benevolent justice was in order. Betty was reluctantly persuaded, but soon she clasped the stand-in to her chest. No matter what the cost, I was glad Baby was back on the bosom of her rightful mother. And then I had to question myself. Who was I fooling? *I* was Mary's baby. I turned to Mom, trying to clear up any confusion. "Mom, you are the best mother in the world."

Mom smiled and looked up at me with adoration. "No, I'm *your* baby!"

I carefully tucked Baby under the blanket on Mom's lap. I hoped no one else had witnessed my infant snatching, yet sometimes it was hard to tell who was a resident and who was a family member or even a new caregiver. The previous week a tall man had approached me, "Do you know where the altar cloth is stored? I'm the priest, and I'm scheduled to serve communion in a few minutes."

"The altar cloth will be found," I'd told him in the patient, articulated tone I used for the memory-care bunch. He wandered down the hall. It wasn't until later that Maria, hurrying by, asked, "Have you see the priest? Some of the residents are waiting for Mass."

I kept a pretty regular schedule to see Mom, and Rosemary brought Celia at least once a week. Residents as well as caregivers were part of our daily lives. There was Ardys, the woman always in crisis about something (we contemplated what a drama her marriage must have been). She constantly hollered from her wheelchair: "But I MUST speak to a gentleman NOW!" her credibility compromised by the fact that she was wearing only an oversize pair of pink long johns. I smiled and waved, walking Mom and Baby to the dining room. Mom's place was set up next to her friend Lainie's as usual, complete with clean bib. Usually I sat with Mom and helped her with the difficult task of spearing chunks of meat or potatoes and getting them safely to her mouth. That night, however, the dining room was understaffed, and I skimmed around the room offering a spoon to Mr. Chu and cutting up chicken for Bunny, who thanked me profusely, then forgot she was supposed to eat. In her former life, Bunny must have been a socialite of some kind, for her mannerisms had that sweater-set cheerfulness possessed by women who hosted myriad, seemingly effortless parties.

"Bye, Bunny!" I said as she headed out of the dining room. She came back, tapped my shoulder, then leaned in and said in a stage whisper, "I just don't know how many people I served tonight." Then with a conspiratorial giggle, "And I'm not even sure what it was I served."

"Oh, it was marvelous!" I reassured her. "Everyone thought it was wonderful." Pleased with herself, she smiled, closed her eyes, and waved her hand behind her ear as if to say, "Oh, it was nothing, really!" and walked off toward her next gala.

I slipped back into my chair next to Mom. "How're you doing here, Mom?"

"Oh, fine fine fine fine," she said and stabbed her finger at the iceberg lettuce smeared with Thousand Island dressing. Then she stopped eating and looked at me, her eyes asking for something deeper. I met her gaze. "You're happy here, aren't you, Mom?"

"Heavens yes yes yes yes."

Amidst clanging spoons and dripping chins, I realized something I hadn't before: Mom was still living her life. Not the life she "*should* be living" or one "disease-free!" but she was surely living it. And it was free of Dad's worry and responsibility. And for the first time in her life she wasn't thinking about making the next meal. She no longer had to please anyone or achieve anything; she just had to be. Her eternal search for the Empty Calendar was over. Here at St. Mont Park she was allowed to throw off the shackles of obligation and revel in a spate of blank calendar days.

Chapter 34.

ᕮ*Beginnings*ᕮ

SHAKESPEARE'S TRAGEDIES INEVITABLY END IN death and destruction. Hamlet lies bloody on the stage; Macbeth is murdered by Macduff; and Othello, obsessed by paranoia, finally kills himself. In other words, the pony dies. Shakespeare's comedies, on the other hand, are usually resolved not in bloody death, but in a wedding. Ole and I chose the latter. After losing Olav, we couldn't picture being apart, as if our baby's brief purpose was to cleave our lives together. In the few years we'd been a couple, we'd also lost both our fathers, Ole's two cats, and one mother was still wandering in the Land of Forgetting. Yet we were determined not to frame our lives as a tragedy. *As You Like It* came to mind, or *All's Well That Ends Well* seemed more appealing.

We sat by the woodstove in the tiny cottage and plotted a story rife with beginnings instead of endings. With the help of Dad's deathbed gift and another from Ole's mom, we'd purchased a small piece of property just a block inland from the cottage, adjacent to the house where Ole had lived when we met. After a year of meeting with an architectural designer, we'd turned our scribblings into plans. The groundbreaking was to take place just weeks after our Memorial Day wedding. For the first time in my life, I was actually putting aside my longtime reservations and preconceptions about marriage and home ownership. In junior high, when many girls were wearing hot pants and loads of makeup, my mother would say ironically, "Too much too soon!" Well, at 49 I certainly wasn't guilty of marrying too soon. Yes, I'd wanted to marry Trey, but as I looked back it was an eyes-closed-I'm-going-to-jump kind of impulse. Rosemary's dictum after I'd returned from Riojos stayed with me: "I'd rather have a man I can live with rather than one I can't live without."

Also, I believed—and Ole did, too—that our wedding warranted some liturgical ballast. There is, after all, beauty in form. Sacraments frame the moments of our lives we cannot fully understand. Birth. Leaving Childhood for Adulthood. Healing. Marriage. Death. In our culture it seems we have dropped most of these ceremonies altogether and marriage often struggles to become the Big Ritual when in fact it has become a cartoon, staggering under the weight of its unrealistic promises.

Ole generously agreed to the 100+ guest list (a public person he is not). He even suggested the venue: the old Victorian theater in our little town, converted into a movie house. The party venue? The bar and restaurant where I'd first played jazz when I arrived in town and the very place Ole and I'd had our first date. We asked our friends in the same combo to provide music for the party. Thanks to the theater proprietor, we sent tickets in the invitations to be presented at the door. And we had a movie poster made, too, with Ole—bow in hand—playing me like a cello. A quotation from Hamlet said, "You can fret me, but you cannot play upon me." The title of the show? *The Wedding*, of course.

Planning a wedding is no small matter. Not only the agony of the guest list (How *many* of the bowmakers should come? Which Norwegian relatives should we choose from Ole's mother's list? What about the caterer's helper who said she wouldn't come if her ex was invited?), but also the logistics of hotels for friends and even the way the historic stage would be set up for the ceremony. And what would I wear instead of the dreaded white gown? I wanted my wedding to be the complete opposite of what I'd always disliked about weddings—stiff, dumb dresses, saccharine vows, sappy toasts, and badly lit reception rooms with guests looking either lost or drunk.

My father's spirit informed my wedding plans, too. I could hear him saying, "Why not!?!" when I suggested to Ole that we might have someone ring the bell in the historic bell tower above town just as the guests came out of the theater after the wedding. It's exactly what my father would have done. As Ole would say, "You always like a parade, Christine."

During the months of planning I'd stop and say to myself, "I am planning my wedding. Am I really using words like bridesmaid and catering?" Luckily I'd had a few gigs teaching at the Navy that spring, and Ole had sold a couple of bows to a prominent quartet, so we had a little extra cash to cover things like the catering. Paul and Rosemary generously chipped in for the wine. Haas assumed the role of wine steward. "I'm thinking a Washington Cab-Sav. It will go well with the salmon, along with a Pinot Gris for those who don't drink red," he said. Haas, the master of making everything sound as if you were in on a secret, a special delight only you and he were privy to.

When our friend Sarah, a gourmet baker who, as a huge gift to us, made our wedding cake, asked, "When are you planning to cut the cake?" I couldn't answer. I was too embarrassed, picturing brides with garters lifting a spatula to push white frosting into their new husband's mouth. My tomboy self was rolling her eyes.

On the other hand, the excitement in my friends and family countered these private moments of hesitation. I was thrilled about Sarah's chocolate hazelnut cake. My ceramist friend Anne offered to design the table setting and flowers. She also suggested using her huge clay tulip vases to grace the bare theater stage during the ceremony. Poets and musicians were to perform at the reception, and the jazz combo would provide the dance music. Another friend would set up a table and two chairs and balloons on the vacant lot where our new house was to be built, and following the next day's picnic people could picture our new house in the making. Since so many had given us wedding presents of doorknobs and light fixtures, coat hooks and hinges, it felt as if everyone were helping us not only start a marriage, but a home as well.

Sas was coming early from Berkeley to help with everything from table setup to getting me dressed for the big moment. "It takes a *village* to get you married off!" Sas said. The fervor of my friends' involvement choked me up. How could I deserve not only Ole, but the love and cheering of so many people I loved? Ole was right. It was a parade.

As far as the ceremony was concerned, I figured I could do what Shakespeare did: write a play within a play. In rhymed couplets, no less. I stole lines from Shakespeare's stories and then wove in a narrative about a "Bowet and a Poet." Smack dab in the middle was the Episcopal Liturgy for Marriage. Our friend Rob, an Episcopal priest and my friend Polly's husband, was chosen to do the honors.

The night before the big day, I drove to St. Mont Park.

"Mom," I said, snuggling next to her on her bed. "I'm getting married tomorrow." I smoothed her hand. She beamed. I didn't know if she understood. Two years after Dad's death, her Renaissance had faded to Baroque. She was mostly in her bed again and could no longer feed herself, but her smile was intact, and she was neither comatose nor unhappy. I believed that she would be there (on some plane) with Ole and me at the theater the next day. I unpacked my wedding outfit and held it up for her to see. A slim, pale celery-green, full-length skirt that flared slightly at the bottom. The fabric shimmered. I held it up to my waist.

"Ooooooo," Mom said and smiled.

Then I held up the black, form-fitting asymmetrical jersey with one long sleeve, the bodice tightly angled across my right breast revealing my bare arm and shoulder. The one long sleeve ended in a graceful bloom around my wrist.

"Yes yes yes yes," Mom fiddled with the bedclothes.

"And look, Mom." I held her own string of pearls up to my neck. "Better late than never, right?" and I laughed, which always elicited a laugh from her. I pulled the high heels out of the bag—black patent leather slingbacks with a slender heel that lifted me high enough to let that satin skirt swish.

Mom smiled again. "Pup pup pup pup…," her gibberish clear in the sound of sense. I had her blessing.

Chapter 35.

❧Built to Last❧

AFTER YEARS OF PACKING MY toolbelt to work on other people's houses, I was finally getting one of my own. No longer was I a laborer while owners leaned over plans, trying to decide where the window should go. Now I was the owner, a wife(!) suggesting if we just might be able to fit a central vacuum system into the budget. I watched while other carpenters hefted rafters and attached clapboard in the southerly winds. Even though Ole and I would do most of the indoor painting, and Ole would lay tile as well as design and install the kitchen, we were not the primary builders. We watched joyously and anxiously as our 1,400-square-foot house grew from the ground up, and the geese flew in Vs over our heads.

Building a house forced Ole and me to think carefully about how we wanted to live, both day to day and in the world. Were we going to indulge in a dishwasher? What about radiant heat? Did it take too much power, or would our southern exposure create enough passive solar to make up for not installing a propane stove?

We did install the vacuum, but we also plumbed for eventual solar hot water, and we had a Rumford fireplace installed for additional heat. As we came into the final stretch, we were exhausted and out of funds. One night at 10:00 p.m. after finally installing the last tile of Marmoleum in the pantry, Ole and I sprawled on the living room floor and wondered if we were going to make it till the end of this project. We'd had to make changes along the way. Our builder Michael had to rein us in on the cost of doors and the front porch. All the choices reminded me of those weekender Vermont clients and how we carpenters would roll our eyes when the owners couldn't decide between a Jotul or a Vermont Castings stove or what kind of lighting to have in their walk-in closet.

Now my own choices seemed equally absurd when viewed in the context of the world's troubles. How could I obsess about choosing between "bronze" and "stainless" finish for the bathroom faucet when more than a billion people across the globe lacked access to clean drinking water? When war-torn families were forced to flee their homes and countries daily?

"How can we justify this?" I asked Ole. "Even if we're building a very small house?"

Ole stood next to the rough-cut slab of cypress that our builder Michael had given us for our kitchen counter and smoothed his hand along the grain.

"Beauty," he said quietly. "We may not be building the perfect house, but we are leaving behind something beautiful, well made. Something built to last."

He was right. One hundred years from now, long after Ole and I have turned to dust, we hoped the occupants of our little house would be gladdened by this well-made structure.

Everything about our home seemed to suggest safety and simplicity. The dormer windows were slanted in proportion to the pitch of the roof, and the arched gate of the courtyard echoed the curve of the rafter tails, ready for clematis and yellow rose to climb over it. Inside the house, we'd built a private nook under the stairs, just big enough for a bookshelf and a cozy bed on the floor for Celia. Our fireplace was constructed of stone from nearby Vancouver Island, the mantel a rough slab laid on top of the supporting stones like a druidic monument. And Ole designed a sitting stone that jutted out from the hearth, for cozying up to the fire. Even the cat doors were framed with Douglas fir trim, so Badger and Callie could have their own swishy, private entrances. The red-clad casement windows and French doors looked great against the oiled cedar clapboards. The French doors opened onto a courtyard where we dreamed of planting fruit trees and roses. Ole's shop was built perpendicular to the house, creating privacy from the road. My little red board-and-batten studio sat opposite the house.

One afternoon before the house was finished, Haas and I sat on the beach. He told me that he was going to Beirut to help start a Lebanese travel magazine. He blinked his impossibly expressive eyes, the dark brown blending into the black, thick lashes. He also showed me a screenplay about a plane crash that involved a lost father. Haas's stories always involved a lost father; his own had died just a month before he was born. Haas had been especially fond of my dad. They'd discussed airlines and time zones and the remote places each had been. After Dad left on his Final Trip, Haas had wept openly. Since our friend was leaving for Beirut, Ole and I delayed our big housewarming for November, when he was due home.

Meanwhile, Ole and I assembled a time capsule to bury in the walls before the sheet-rockers finished. In a large plastic tube we stuffed a copy of our daily *New York Times*, a *New Yorker* magazine, and the recent issue of our local newspaper. We included our house plans, our wedding invitation tube, and photos of Ole's bows played by musicians around the globe. I slipped in a couple of poems, too, hoping that down the road those words might still inspire someone. If they failed to do so, we also tucked in a bottle of Washington State wine.

We moved in on my fiftieth birthday in mid-July. That morning, preparing for the stacks of boxes due to arrive, I'd swept the floor of the woodshop next to Ole's bowmaking studio. When I scooshed the last pile into the dustpan, something stuck out among the shavings and dirt: it turned out to be one of the miniature falconry bell earrings that Trey had given me for my birthday back in Riojos. I was baffled. I was certain I'd left them in Riojos, but there it was, its partner gone the way of lost things, the gold bell crushed beyond tinkling, the feathery tail twisted. I swept it into the pan.

One day shortly after we'd moved in, our neighbor Fred slowed his pickup just as I was carrying groceries into the house.

"Want to buy a horse?" he said, leaning out the window and inching his brown Ford pickup onto the shoulder.

"What?" I stopped in my tracks, shifting my bag of vegetables onto my other hip. "That little Arabian?" I remembered the flashy way that horse moved, as if he had a plan and his spirit was moving toward it.

"Yup," Fred said.

"Why?" I set down my bag on the step.

"I just don't have enough time for him these days. He needs work and activity. He's smart and I just can't be with him as I'd like to." I pictured that sleek gelding getting fat and sassy on the summer grass.

"He's a great horse," Fred said. "You'll never find another like him."

"What's his name?" I asked.

"Buddy," Fred said.

"Kind of an inauspicious name for such a beautiful horse…"

"He came with the name."

"Oh, Fred," I sighed. "It's not an option right now. Ole and I just moved in. It cost a lot more than we thought it would, building this little place." We both looked up at the house, the shapely curve of the chimney.

"Well. You think about it," Fred said, turning his truck back onto the road. "I have a good monthly deal on the pasture on Henry Street. We could split the rent. My mules are there, too."

I stuffed that possibility back down as far as it could go, glad that the gelding was still pastured where I could not see him. The news unnerved me. Not only was that horse beautiful, he was available. I couldn't open that door again. It was too big, too freighted with emotion, time, and money. Especially after Ole and I had spent every ounce of our energy finishing this house. I knew what it took to keep a horse, and it was more than hay and grain.

I swung the groceries onto my other hip, went inside, and shut the door.

Chapter 36.

⟷ *Down in the River to Pray* ⟷

ON CHRISTMAS EVE, ROSEMARY WHEELED Mom out of her room to the big decorated tree in the St. Mont Park lobby. Muzak was piping the same arrangements of carols we'd heard year after year, the crèche was in the same place on the piano, and the familiar quilted reindeer draped over the chairs. Unlike our family traditions when I was a child (such as the annual washing and pressing of all the doll clothes and arranging every single one of our stuffed animals and dolls on the settee to wait for Santa), St. Mont Park's Christmas felt like an old video loop. I even recognized the pretend wrapped presents under the tree. Mom had been living at St. Mont Park for five years.

Sitting there in the festooned room, "Silent Night" playing for the hundredth time, Rosemary reached over to Mom's forearm, limp on the wheelchair hand rest.

"Mom, don't you think it's time to press on now? Don't you want to go and join Dad? It's okay if you do. We're ready, too. Christine is married now. She has her own house. You are free to go!" Rosemary and I laughed, along with Mom, knowing it was exactly the kind of thing she would have agreed to.

In fact, she did. One week later, an unexpected infection was coursing through Mom's body, and the doctor said it would not be much longer for her; her vital signs were weak. In Mom's directives, she had not wanted to be kept alive under these circumstances, something Dad had made clear when she moved to St. Mont Park. It's a touchy subject, of course, and most every family has to navigate through it. In her cogent life, Mom had always been decisive about such things ("The Hemlock Society makes sense!"), and, while Dad strode straight toward the Other Side, Mom trod more softly. By New Year's Eve, Paul was flying back to Seattle on a red-eye.

Rosemary and I met at St. Mont Park, prepared to spend the night. I'd brought a bottle of champagne, but Rosemary said she was too tired and went across the hall to sleep in an empty resident room. The little Christmas tree Rosemary had set up for Mom on her first St. Mont Park Christmas glowed on the windowsill. Outside, snow and sleet came down in guttural breaths, spitting against the window. I sat with Mom in the dark. At the stroke of midnight, boat horns tooted in the harbor, and sodden fireworks drooped across a wet sky.

"Oh, heck, Mom," I said and turned on the light. "Let's have that champagne."

Mom breathed and made a tiny squeak. I took a couple of tiny, plastic medicine cups from the cupboard, a towel from her sink, and opened that bottle of Brut.

"Happy New Year, Mom," I said and tipped back the urine-sample-sized vessel. I held her cup to her lips, and she made little sipping sounds. And then I put the cups down, side by side. Out the window in the dark harbor, the horns subsided, and I lay down in my nest bed on the floor.

With Paul's arrival the next morning, Mom's face lit up. "Oooohhhhhh!" she said, something she hadn't done in a long time. Clearly, out of the fog she recognized Paul. "Hi, Mommykins," Paul said and held her hand. Having all three children there seemed to make her safe and ready, to finally get on with it. Within a day she was semiconscious.

We sat around Mom's bed and sang three-part harmonies for her. We revived old Episcopal chestnuts like "All Things Bright and Beautiful" to spirituals like "Swing Low, Sweet Chariot," and then our favorite, a tune from the movie *Oh, Brother, Where Art Thou?* titled "Down in the River and Pray," one we'd actually worked on the previous week when he and his girls had been out for Christmas. Paul could get that bass moving, and Rosemary took over soprano. We sang and sang and sang.

"When will Mom become Not Mom?" I asked Rosemary as we unfolded the Scrabble board.

"I don't know, but this is big," she said. "We only have two parents. This only happens twice. So, this is it." She labeled our score sheet "The Scrabble Death Watch."

My siblings and I wondered who might gather around our own death beds. I veered away from contemplating the absence of my three unborn children, but like a radar Rosemary read my thoughts and said, "Oh, Christine, you'll have hundreds of friends gathering around you. Including all our girls. People will be taking numbers. Playing tunes and reading poems. *Your* poems, of course…It will be a *spectacle*." She folded the blanket at the foot of Mom's bed and patted Mom's feet.

Finally, Rosemary said, "I'm hungry." Paul agreed, "We should head out for some quick dinner, don't you think?" I put on my coat. Before leaving the room, I looked over at Mom breathing quietly, her hair like a crooked halo behind her on the pillow.

"I think I'll stay behind," I said. "Would you guys mind bringing back some takeout?" Before Paul and Rosemary left, my Scrabble score hovered at 87 while Rosemary's hit 103. This was fairly early in the game, and we always played for broke. With my siblings gone, I quietly brushed Mom's hair, then climbed right in bed with her and held her. Her head lay on my shoulder and her breath got quieter and she inhaled in tiny sips like bird breaths.

"I love you, Mom," I said. "Everything's going to be okay." I smoothed the blanket and said a quiet prayer for her safe and easy journey.

"Hey! We've got pizza, lasagna, and beer," Paul, laden with bags, appeared in the doorway. We pushed aside the Scrabble game and perched on our chairs around Mom. On my second bite of lasagna, Mom's cheeks started to turn white as her breath came in tiny teaspoonfuls. I laid my plate on the floor.

"This is it, you guys," I said. "Mom's going now," and moved toward her as if to help her on her way. Paul put down his plate and actually moved away, as if to give her room to leave. Rosemary just began to sing. In a deep, strong voice, her music filled the room, "*Into thy hands, oh, Lord/ We commend thy spirit...*" Rosemary's anthem came from a familiar and comforting place. No longer were we sitting with the smell of pizza and death in a small room in the House of Forgetting. We were home again, safe with Mom and Dad, our old upright piano plankety-planking out the songs of childhood.

"We love you, Mom," I said, and we all waved, as if she could see us as she left her body. As with Dad, I looked up to see if I could see her spirit rise. For ten years she'd endured this mysterious disease; I felt a lightness in the room, a release.

"No more Alzheimer's, Mom!" I said, when her breath finally stopped.

"Wahoo," Paul said. "You made it, Mom."

We kept the door closed and sat with Mom long after she'd gone, singing more hymns, talking about the family, and contemplating the state of orphanhood.

"Our parents *always* die in January," Rosemary said.

"Well, you were the one who killed Mom," Paul pointed at Rosemary. "Telling her to go!"

"Not to mention *Dad,*" Rosemary admitted, reminding us that it had been she who'd offered Dad the option of hospice, something neither Paul nor I could bear to do.

But Rosemary came back with a left hook. "I could do that for them, though…because Mom and Dad liked me best."

"Ohhh, no," Paul chimed in, taking a sip of his beer. Mom's face grew whiter and whiter. "I was the shining star, their first child! I knew they liked *me* best."

"I hate to disappoint you guys," I turned my chair away from Mom to face my siblings. "I was the *fun* one! They liked me best because I was funny. I might have been the *bad* one, the one they worried about most, but they knew I was worth it. I was their favorite. Like the prodigal son!" Mom's limbs got stiffer, jaw dropping, her hair wild.

We kept the door locked for over an hour before reporting her death to the authorities at St. Mont Park—so Mom wouldn't be rushed, so she could take her own time to leave the party. We toasted our mother, but I was also toasting something else. My experience with these deaths had been many things, but fear was not among them. As I looked around the room at my brother and sister fully embodied in the flesh and my mother transformed beyond it, I was struck by what my parents had given me. Not only my life, but in their dying, they'd given me courage to face the fear of death.

I could almost see Mom sitting at our kitchen table in Meadowdale, smiling and smoothing the tablecloth with her hands, her gold wedding band making that familiar click on the table. In her let's-go-over-the-details voice, she was laughing, "Now wasn't that a dumb thing I had there, toward the end?"

Chapter 37.

❧Things Temporal and Eternal❧

MORNING SUN PLAYED WITH THE surface of the pond across from Ole's and my new house. Violet-green swallows swooped and dived toward the birdhouses Ole had made, anticipating their arrival almost to the day. The flower box he built for our bedroom window tumbled with sweet alyssum, blue lobelia, and pansies. Yellow roses were beginning their climb over our courtyard gate.

I stood at the mailbox, looking back at our new house, which seemed as if it had always been planted there among the firs. In the nine short months since we'd moved in, that little house had learned quickly how to accommodate absence. My mother's memorial had stretched the house's walls just eight weeks before, yes, but our first real housewarming party had turned out to be a memorial, too. Haas had sent me an email from Lebanon, with flight numbers and arrival times for our big party, planned both as a celebration of our house and his homecoming. *"We'll soon be sitting sipping a glass of wine! Having WILD salmon,"* he wrote. *"So much to tell you! The 10-hour time difference is not helping matters…I will try to call you Friday night my time. You'll be busy making the Halloween costume for Celia Rose! Wonder what she'll be this year!?XXX"*

Haas never called that Friday, nor did he return from Beirut. The day after I received this email, his heart stopped. He and his new boyfriend were just about to have dinner. The wine was cold, the fish warm. It was as if he'd stepped out to look at the stars and never came back. I still expected him to drive into our driveway, leap out of his red truck, and wave a bottle of champagne.

Our house had carried a lot in its short life. I was especially glad for its welcoming windows and its safe, protective walls. I would need them.

As I returned from the mailbox, my neighbor Fred slowed his Ford pickup and rolled down the window. For the second time—in less than a year—he asked if I'd like to buy that horse of his, the one named Buddy.

"Oh, Fred…," I said. The June sunlight reflected off the cab of the truck, rays bouncing off the rearview mirror. "Actually, uh, I can't really think about that right now…" The absurdity of his timing hit me all at once. I clutched the mail, wondering whether I could tell Fred what I'd been told in a darkened room the day before. I was still in shock myself, barely able to wrap my mind around yet another sudden turn in my life. Does one just blurt out to your neighbor (a gruff one, no less?) that you've been diagnosed with breast cancer? How depressing is that? I gave it a try.

Fred's face dropped, and I could tell he didn't know what to say. He opened the door, stepped out, and hugged me hard, holding extra-long, then jumped back into his truck. Before he pulled away, a singular impulse shot through me, and, as if grabbing the golden ring on a merry-go-round, I lifted my hand, "Wait!! Fred!" He braked and let the truck idle.

"On second thought," I said, "…it just occurred to me. I mean it looks like I may be out of commission for a while. The doctor says it could be months to a year. Surgery, radiation, and maybe chemo, depending…We actually don't know yet." Fred's face was somber.

"Even though Ole and I can't *buy* Buddy, would it be okay—I mean— if I went over to his meadow? To work with him a little?"

I didn't know what I'd do with that horse—I didn't even know how I'd be feeling—but it seemed to make sense. Just to go see a horse.

"Well, of course." Fred was clearly glad to have something to say. "Any time. Buddy's in the big field at the end of Henry Street. You'll see the mules, too. Molly and Gracie. They're all there." Fred gave me a long look, then pulled away.

It had all happened so fast. One day I'm planting lavender in our new courtyard, preparing for Ole's and my wedding anniversary, the next day I find a strange pucker in my right breast and I'm on a conveyor belt toward the Unknown. My local doctor wasn't happy with what she felt in the examination (my annual mammogram had revealed nothing unusual, and I'd had a physical only a month or so before), so she immediately made an appointment for advanced 3-D imaging at a hospital an hour away on the Peninsula. The problem was, they couldn't fit me in until after the Memorial Day weekend. Ole and I spent our anniversary barely sipping pale ale at a café, clutching hands underneath the table.

When Tuesday finally came, my nerves had tangled into a tight coil of distress. Ole bought some valerian root pills, a natural sedative, and I popped two before we drove to the high-tech mammogram, but it didn't seem to make any difference.

Even before they took images of my breasts, nurses chirped, "Don't worry! You can get new breasts! Reconstruction is totally possible!!" When the doctor pointed to my mammogram blazing from the monitor, her face told Ole and me everything. "How long have you had *that?*" the doctor said, her accusatory finger on what appeared to be a dark mass in my right breast. "You might have it in both breasts, actually. You need a biopsy right away. If I were you, I'd go to the front desk and make an appointment with a surgeon." Her appalling bedside manner punctured my thin veneer of calm. My husband wrapped his arm around me, escorted me right out of that room, and we drove home.

I called Rosemary immediately.

"Don't make an appointment at that hospital," she said. "I'm calling Dr. Kara Carlson at Evergreen right now." Apparently, Rosemary knew a diagnostic radiologist at the healthcare facility where she contracted as a freelance publicist and video producer. She said one wing was devoted specifically to breast health. Dr. Carlson was able to see me the next day. Rosemary would meet us there. The conveyor belt was picking up speed.

As we made the familiar half-hour ferry crossing, Ole and I stood on the breezy deck knowing our lives had already changed course. With the losses racking up, we were facing them as one; we were family now. But in my vulnerable state, I deeply missed my mother. She would know the right thing to say about this new development. A phrase or a quip that would make it all less dire, less furrowed brow. Mt. Rainier loomed over the Seattle skyline, and the Cascades rose like pure white teeth across the Sound.

I was greeted at the hospital by a friendly nurse who escorted me to the biopsy room. "How are you feeling today?" she asked quietly. I did not tell her that my stomach was writhing in knots, that my parents were dead, that my darling friend was also dead, that I'd hardly eaten for days, and that every object (even the warm gown she offered me) felt like a harbinger of doom.

After the biopsy, Rosemary, Ole, and I were taken into a darkened consulting room with comfy chairs and soft blue carpeting. There were whiteboards and screens, but Dr. Carlson offered us a seat and got right to it. "Well, yes," she said, "you do have cancer." Collective intake of breath. "But from what it looks like now it may be slow-growing."

We all brightened slightly in spite of ourselves (was this good news?).

"Then she won't have to lose her breast?" Rosemary's voice rose and held like a C-major chord.

Dr. Carlson looked directly at me and crossed her shapely legs. "I'm afraid you will" (bad news). "We found not one, but two cancerous tumors in there. Considering where they are located, combined with the size of your breast, we would not be able to save it" (bad news, definitely bad). Addressing all three of us, Dr. Carlson said, "We will do an MRI to make sure there is nothing in the other breast. And the surgeon, Dr. Johnson—she'll need that imaging for the surgery. The surgery will reveal if the cancer has progressed into your lymph nodes."

An MRI? Hadn't they already discovered what they needed to know? Was this lovely Dr. Carlson suggesting there was more? (Another point for bad news.)

"But now, the nurse will take you to Dr. Hunter," Dr. Carlson said, as if we were special guests in a private club. "Dr. Hunter is our radiation oncologist and meets with every new patient before she begins her treatment. He will outline your case and tell you what to expect." Dr. Carlson stopped and smiled, "I think you'll like him." Then she touched my arm, "I'm glad you came here. We'll take care of you."

In the course of a few short minutes I had breathed in the worst possible news and then breathed it out. Though I was shaky and vacant (how much adrenaline can the body produce exactly?), suddenly—out of nowhere—my reserve tank kicked in. As if Mom and Dad had opened to door for me, a wave of resolve surged, and, seeing that there was no time to wallow, I rose out of my chair and asked the nurse her name. "Wilma," she said and smiled.

"May I hold your hand, Wilma, on the way to see this Dr. Hunter?"

"Of course," she said and slipped her soft hand into mine. We strode far ahead of Rosemary and Ole toward this alleged Dr. Hunter, and as we turned the corner into Radiation Oncology, the image of Badger came to mind. Instead of running *away* from the coyotes or the dogs who hounded him, he always seemed to walk straight *toward* them. I pretended I was my black-and-white cat with a mustache.

"Welcome!" Dr. Hunter said standing from his huge desk and reaching out his hand to shake mine. He wore a fine tailored suit and tie, his face made all the more radiant by his open, welcoming smile. Wilma disappeared and there we were—Rosemary, Ole, and me, the Three Amigos—in yet another room to discuss the C-word. Dr. Hunter encouraged us all to sit down.

"Judging by what Dr. Carlson has found, I think you may have dodged a bullet here" (good news?). "Of course, surgery will reveal the true nature of this cancer" (bad news) "and whether or not it has made it to your lymph nodes" (unthinkable). After launching into the science of my particular tumor, he explained the statistics of recurrence and relative survival rates of breast cancer with the ease and delight of a baseball fan quoting batting averages. "But you caught this early, which is always a good thing when it comes to breast cancer. We've already put together a team for you."

Rosemary, Ole, and I shared surreptitious glances. Who was this doctor (his skin like the smooth ebony on one of Ole's bows) with perfect recall for numbers, quoting medical cases off the top of his head?

"Yes," he said, registering our surprise, and laughed. "I stay up at night and study this stuff. It's my entertainment!" I pictured this striking man stretched out on a designer sofa, stacks of journals by his side, and maybe a glass of wine on the coffee table, devouring knowledge bite by bite.

"And I might add that the surgeon assigned to you is top level. I would bring my own family to her. We call her 'the artist.' And your medical oncologist, Dr. Klein? She is very quiet, but she is one of the finest cancer doctors in the field. Radically smart. If I had cancer, I'd want to be treated by her." The thought of Dr. Hunter afflicted even with a common cold was unimaginable. His body radiated health and vigor.

And then he asked me what I did for a living. "A poet! Well, we need to keep our poets alive, don't we? I would love to read your work." And when he discovered Ole was a maker of bows for stringed instruments, he shifted into high gear. "I used to collect antique bows!" he said, addressing Ole as if they were colleagues. "Piccattes, Tourtes…the French ones, you know. I had them all. Then I got interested in other things." Those other things turned out to be ballroom dancing, fencing, and learning several languages.

By the end of our meeting my stomach had stopped churning. Yes, I had cancer. And no, they still didn't know how far it had spread or its true nature. But Dr. Hunter had somehow created a picture we could fit into, one that contained a Vermeer window with a thin band of buttery-yellow light filtering in.

When we met "the artist," we knew we were in the right hands. Sporty and direct, Dr. Johnson said that the initial biopsy looked very promising (good news?). She said she didn't foresee finding any stray cells in the lymph nodes. "I'm really hoping you won't have to go through the agony of chemo," she said, her long graceful fingers explaining what the surgery entailed. "But we will know everything after the lymph nodes are biopsied."

As this diagnosis expanded and contracted, I called my friends who'd gone through what I was now calling the Breast Cancer Adventure (BCA). I hoped they could give me some reassuring advice, especially since everything still seemed so up in the air. Even Dr. Hunter's positive meeting paled if I thought too hard about lymph nodes—not to mention the prospect of Dr. Johnson's scalpel poised over my breast. When I called my friend Jo, who'd faced the same treatment, she said, "You'll feel better once you have a plan, Christine. Once you have a strategy, there's a purpose and you'll see—" Jo paused. "This is the hardest part, the not-knowing."

In the days before I was due for surgery, however, there was one thing I did know for sure. I pulled on a pair of brand-new logging boots sent by a friend "for courage." (She'd even gotten my size right.) They were made of supple, black leather with slanted, strong heels, and they laced up high above my ankles in a way that gave me some real mojo. I strode toward the woods where I'd heard there was a shortcut to Bluff Meadows. Curiously, in my years in the neighborhood, I'd never been over there, even though Buddy's field was only a ten-minute walk from our new house.

As I emerged from the trees on that sunny June day and walked the short distance to the pasture gate, I could see chickens scratching near a big barn where barn swallows flew in and out of the sagging door. A breeze blew the tall grass in waves, and I could hear the ocean crashing below the cliff. In the distance a white horse with dapples on his loins grazed with two mules at his side. The wind blew his mane, which revealed a lean and graceful neck. When I neared the gate, he lifted his head and immediately walked briskly toward me, his ears pricked forward as if to say, "Hey! Who are you!? Whassup?"

Waiting for Test Results. These four words are contemporary shorthand for "I am pretending life is normal!" or "Look! I'm walking across the lawn, the very lawn that was here yesterday but today it looks quite different." Or "Don't I seem casual, lying here in my bed with my laptop, waiting for the phone to ring? Actually, my belly feels like a swarm of writhing eels."

Surgery day hadn't been easy. I'd been given breathing practices by my yoga teacher, Noelle, I'd been sent meditation CDs from my friend Belinda in Vermont, and I had prayed. Rosemary's Episcopal minister had even come to bless me before going to the operating room. But soon after I emerged into recovery, they rushed me to the Intensive Care Unit: my heart had decided to rev up into panic mode as a result of dehydration during the operation. (Whose heart wouldn't speed up?)

Dr. Johnson had told Rosemary and Ole, however, that she was very optimistic after removing three "sentinel nodes" from my armpit. She said the tissue had looked clean (good news!). My heart and I were finally discharged, and Ole took me home to recover and await the new results.

Combined with the pain from surgery (my throbbing right side was wrapped in a big bandage), the suspense of not knowing still hovered over that bright sunny day. Ole brought me lemonade in bed, and yet my future—both immediate and long-term—depended on Dr. Johnson's call, that phone on my comforter the conduit of all things temporal and eternal.

Badger and Callie lay next to me, and each time the phone rang I jumped. Every call, however, turned out to be a concerned friend. "No furrowed brow!" I told them. "No leaning in with worry lines on your face. That's my only request."

Just when I thought I couldn't stand the waiting another minute, my brother emailed me via iTunes the first cut of classical singer Susan Graham's CD titled *À Chloris* (the name of a Greek nymph associated with flowers and gardens). I clicked Paul's message, opened the file, and listened to Graham's pure voice as I lay in waiting. Instead of my heart lurching, the music held it as if by an invisible hand.

I played *À Chloris* over and over on my laptop like a mantra. Graham's voice sang the Reynaldo Hahn melody with a tinge of expectation, as if the smells of those flowers from the title surrounded her music. It's the piano, really, that makes that song so poignant. The recurring triplet and then the held-back quarter notes. So tender, but hopeful with a whiff of sorrow. I prayed that the cancer had not strayed to the sweet garden of my lymph nodes, and I played the song over and over and over, trying to will good news into that sunny afternoon. News like Badger and Callie's soft purring next to me. Like the scent of lavender.

Chapter 38.

ᴕ*Purification Rites*ᴕ

Rosemary, Ole, and I stuffed ourselves into the cramped examination room with my quiet oncologist, Dr. Allie Klein. The three of us towered over her, even in our chairs. She perched on a tiny stool, her feet barely touching the ground. She wore a pair of neat little slacks, flat shoes with straps that buckled, and a cardigan sweater. Her short, black hair stuck up straight and shiny with a touch of product.

I'd met her briefly the week before, soon after the Phone Call from Dr. Johnson, who had reported that one of the three "sentinel" lymph nodes she'd removed from my armpit had indeed contained cancer cells. "I'm sorry," Dr. Johnson had said. The day of *À Chloris* wilted, and I nearly squeezed off Ole's hand.

"I so much didn't want to deliver this news," Dr. Johnson told me. "I was thinking it would be otherwise." She sounded as if it were her fault that one sleeping sentinel had failed to deflect the errant cells.

The definitive plan was six months of chemotherapy followed by a month of rest, then several more months of radiation. No worries about how I had to fill my calendar for the next year: my datebook was packed. Initially the diagnosis warranted what was deemed a lighter dose of chemo, except today in this miniature examination room, my oncologist was telling me something else.

"I've spent the week mulling over your case," Dr. Klein said softly, looking directly at me. "I'm not feeling the love about the protocol I originally recommended. I've changed my mind." My heart lurched again, a double shot of adrenaline feeding those eels in my belly. Rosemary clickety-clacked notes onto her laptop, and Ole looked pale. He'd hardly slept, either.

Then Dr. Klein listened intently while I showered her with questions: How long? What will it feel like? What are the side effects again? What are those risks you mentioned? Do I really have to have the big kahuna treatment, really? Her smile, like a tiny parenthesis on its side, turned up when I said, "kahuna."

"I want to blast this," Dr. Klein said calmly, her face unfurrowed but resolved. "You are young and strong. I believe you can handle it." To each question she gave thoughtful and complete answers. Not only that, while I was talking, Dr. Klein took notes on tiny yellow Post-its and carefully stuck them onto the file folder with my name on it.

When Rosemary stopped typing, the room went quiet. Like Ole, this doctor with her calm shoulders and tiny Post-its was comfortable with silence. When I finally said, "Thank you, Dr. Klein," she said, "Call me Allie," and folded her delicate hands in her lap as if she had nowhere else to be but right there in that room with us.

"You can do this," she tells me with quiet authority. "I will be your cheerleader, your guide."

When I see Buddy's curious face coming toward me in the early July sunshine, mules trailing along behind him like attendants—all the fear and trepidation I've sustained in the last month recedes. By now Buddy knows me, and he nickers when he sees me coming. I've introduced him to Ole, and one day when I was there alone, I climbed up on the water trough and slipped onto his back (just to feel his power) then quickly slid down.

He noses my pocket for a carrot and follows me over to a sunny corner of the meadow. I sit down in the shade of a tree. When Gracie and Molly try to stand near me, Buddy flattens his ears, and they step back obediently. Buddy takes up the space next to me and dozes, his ambrosial breath against my neck. Time is irrelevant in the sun-dappled shade, and I have the strange assurance that I am exactly where I need to be.

I do not tell Buddy about my surgery, my first weeks of chemotherapy—my Purification Rites—nor do I mention that my hair is already starting to fall out, how Ole has given me a tightly shorn haircut to prepare for what's to come, how I'd watched hanks of my blonde hair spill onto the bathroom floor. Buddy doesn't have any use for these irrelevant details. He just takes my breath away. And gives it back.

By the end of the month, Ole had removed the remaining clumps of my hair with the vacuum cleaner. He used duct tape to remove the rest. My eyelashes were long gone and so were my eyebrows. Strange how the absence of these punctuation marks rendered my face more vulnerable, but the basic structure remained. I gazed in the mirror at my eyes and cheekbones, which had become more pronounced. "Ole," I said. "I look just like my father. That's my father's face looking back at me."

I could feel my father's spirit accompanying me on the BCA, especially in a purchase Ole and I made shortly after the diagnosis. The thought of nearly a year's cancer treatment on my great-grandmother's cramped antique bed on our old, compressed futon didn't appeal to either of us, so (just as my father would have done) we sprang for a new bed, with something called "Independent Coil Suspension" available on a payment plan. We even bought the cheap sleigh-bed frame. Nothing like a little cancer treatment to inspire home decoration.

Or fashion, for that matter. One day right before the infusion while I was still feeling pretty strong (it ebbed and flowed, that elixir of love), Rosemary, Celia, and I went to the wig room at the Breast Center. The volunteer was still so angry about losing both her breasts to cancer, she could not focus on what Rosemary and I might be looking for. "They took them from me!" she said, her face set. "They were my pride and joy." Right then and there we knew a wig was not what we were after. We beetled over to REI. Veering past the backpacks and ice axes, hiking boots and various Spandex outfits, we found a shelf of bright-colored buffs, headgear that athletes wear as sweat bands, ear muffs, or even neck warmers. We grabbed light-blue ones and another with giraffes, another with National Geographic logos and whales. Celia, prancing down the aisle, spotted a red-and-gray Gortex rain hat that looked like a floppy cowboy hat.

"Hey, Christine!!" Celia jumped up and down. "This might be nice for your bare head!" she said expertly. Rosemary bought everything, and we left with an armful of color.

Surgery was scary enough (a slice of one's body disappearing into the ether?), but as I ventured into Purification Rites, the safe geography of life as I knew it disappeared, and soon I was in a foreign land. Unfamiliar mountains rose up, and the mouths of caves hollered from the dark wood. They say you must do such things on your own. And I did, but I discovered there were attendants everywhere, just waiting to help me step over the hot lava and dark chasms, to hold my hand when I was blind with distress. And they always seemed to show up at just the right time. Ole and Rosemary were my constants, of course, and my close friends were beyond stellar with meals and moral support, but also there was the ferry toll booth guy who ushered our car to the head of the line, so we wouldn't have to wait for the next boat home. Or Valerie, who asked no fee for gentle bodywork sessions at my home. I never knew when she left, since I was sound asleep. And one morning, I looked out my bedroom window to see our neighbor Fred mowing our lawn.

Also, the hospital—the very site of my fears—housed some of my most ardent comforters: Stephen, the nurse who found a fan to keep me cool in postsurgery discomfort. My oncology nurse, Kris, whose hands were gentle as swan's wings. I wept the moment I saw her coming, my fear assuaged by her soft words, her generous body, her smile, the little cross she wore around her neck; when I gave myself over to loving her, the fear stepped back. Jen, Dr. Allie's assistant, always met me with a smile and a gesture of normalcy like, "How do you like my new haircut? I gave everything to Locks of Love!" Patrick, the young man who drew my blood, loved talking about his son Evan, whom he was raising alone. When I asked him about Evan's birthday party, the world seemed to switch back in balance. These people became my family, and kindness was the primary currency. I was swimming in a bath of tender mercies. I even sang to Kris each time I returned to the Font: *"Ol' Man Chemo, Ol' Man Chemo…He must know somethin' but he don't say nothin'. He just keeps rollin', he keeps on rollin' along…"*

So, as Purification rolled on, the infusion room at Evergreen became a kind of temple, and I remembered that my friend Sawnie, who had suffered for years with acute chronic fatigue, had told me that all illness is a form of healing. That helped me weather out the three days after the infusion on Rosemary's deck, and at night in her big guest bed. I quickly discovered that thinking isn't really all it's cracked up to be. It just gets in the way. Purification was a no-brain experience. My mind took a backseat to the feelingness of things. When I needed a retreat from the agony, I'd imagine

Buddy and his cute ears pointed delicately inward and the way he stamped his foot at the gate when I came to see him.

In one particularly grueling post-Font night at Rosemary's, I'd lain awake for hours, wanting to crawl out of my body and be rid of the thunder and lightning inside of me, a wounded animal just trying to find a cave. The trouble was, there was no safe cave. My body was a husk I wanted to crawl *out* of. Then, right in the middle of my Sturm und Drang, outside the window a tree frog began his raspy soliloquy. Though every inch of me wanted to leave my skin, the tree frog zapped me right back into creation. *He* wasn't concerned about my distress. But then he wasn't *un*concerned, either. The frog's voice came through that open window with such confidence and clarity I found myself calling back to him, "Thankyouthankyouthankyouthankyouthankyouthankyou-thankyou."

Chapter 39.

⮑ *Port of Good Hope* ⮐

AFTER THE FONT—AND THE DAYS after when I often stayed on at Rosemary's—I felt like Hamlet's Uncle Claudius describing Hamlet: "Like the hectic in my blood he rages!" Even my teeth ached. The irony, however, was baldly evident: I wanted to treatment to be over, yet I was receiving it to *extend life*. Hurry up and live?

I sweated and tossed in Rosemary's guest bed, groping for a thought or prayer to calm me, a cheery image to get me through.

Buddy.

Even saying his name seemed to push away the fear and dread. One night I turned on the light, grabbed my laptop, and googled "Arabian horse." Immediately I was captured by a YouTube video that opened with evocative Arabic music. A man in a white robe and turban puts on a pair of Ray-Bans. Behind him, through the aisle of the barn, trots a dazzling bay Arabian stallion, free—without constraint. The horse noses the smiling, gentle Bedouin, and the video cuts to a huge sandy arena, beyond which stretches the wide-open desert. The horse gallops in delight, its tail up high.

When the man holds up his arms and raises his crop, the horse gallops toward him, then stops and rears, pawing at the startling, blue sky. The Bedouin races down the middle of the arena, robes flowing, and the stallion trots along beside him like a dog. The video cuts again to a pedestal in the middle of the arena, and the man mysteriously beckons the stallion from the far end. The horse races toward the pedestal and comes to a graceful halt, placing his front feet squarely on the box. The man (Who is he? The titles are all in Arabic) rubs the horse's neck and turns, smiling, to the camera. I watched that YouTube video at least six times before getting to sleep, and many times after that, night after night. What was this magical dance of gentleness and joy? I wanted it. The taste of desire vanquished the bitter cup of chemo.

By my birthday in July, I couldn't focus my eyes. ("Chemo-brain!" Dr. Hunter told me). Ole cut his hair in a buzz cut in deference to my head, and Rosemary gave me a beautiful red French butter dish. Celia gave me Chapstick. The vision thing was weird, though. It was too much stimuli even to watch a movie, and all I could do was surrender to my body (surrender being much different from giving in). "A.C," Adriamycin and Cytoxan, the duo firebrands coursing through my veins, sounded like characters from Greek myth. This protocol was indeed the big kahuna. I counted the days till I would switch to Taxol in the fall, which was supposed to be less harrowing.

Luckily, during the initial surgery, Dr. Johnson had inserted a "port" so that each time I came to the Font, Kris didn't have to insert a needle in my arm. The little round entry looked like a plastic bottle cap. I called it "The Port of Good Hope." Since I couldn't see to read, after dinner Ole would read aloud to me. It became a nightly bright spot. We'd finished Ivan Doig's *The Sea Runners*, and we were on to *The Life of Pi*, about a boy stranded in a boat in the middle of the ocean with a Bengal tiger. He doesn't know where he is going. He, too, needed a Port of Good Hope.

One rainy morning when Ole was out working in his shop, a man in a black suit appeared at the front door with literature for what he called "The Last Day."

"Thank you," I tell him, eager to return to my couch, "but I'm on my own path."

"Oh," he says, checking out my blue REI buff headgear he clearly links with infidels. "Does your religion know about the End?"

I assure him that I know a bit about that, yes…(Should I tell him that the Kingdom of God is not off in the future, bound by dogma? Shall I let him know I am learning daily that any kingdom we share exists only in this moment and is ultimately only about love?)

The man's mouth is pressed tight and turned down in worry, but I assure him I am in the right hands, that he need not fret.

"Watch the slippery step," I tell him as he turns to leave.

Later I stagger over to Buddy's field. He comes over to sniff my boots, and we walk around the damp meadow, him following me. I find his halter hanging on a nail in the barn (baby swallows peeping!) and slip it over his graceful head. He has such a big spirit, I'd hardly noticed he was less than fifteen hands tall. I urge him to circle me at the end of the lead, but he feints left, then tosses his head as if to say, "Whee! Watch me! I'm Little Big Man!"

When I'd asked Dr. Allie if it was okay to play with a horse, she'd hesitated, tipped her head, and said, "A horse?" I explained about my new friend and how he whinnied when he saw me coming. She smiled her little parenthesis smile and said, "Just be careful. Your immune system is compromised right now, so you don't want him to step on you or anything; you don't want to risk infection." Her eyebrows went up. "But I don't see anything wrong with having a friend…"

When Buddy trots around me in the meadow, I forget the hectic in my blood, and I revel in the lines of this horse. And who knew that the smell of horse would seduce me again? Buddy's hide, his flesh, his breath, his neck where I bury my face? He comes to a halt and looks directly at me, his white eyelashes long and expressive, it feels as if I've known him from somewhere before. My mother would be dazzled by this horse. She'd see that little twinkle of mischief in his eyes and laugh, too. I wonder if she has anything to do with this horse prancing into my dark days. Not a moment too soon.

One morning I got out of the tub, and Ole cupped my left breast in his hand. "This breast is working for two," he said, kissed it, then handed me a towel. I had to hand it to Dr. Johnson; she was an artist: Her surgical line was elegant. And not gory at all. A smooth, graceful desert where one small hill used to stand. Absence becoming presence, like negative space in a painting. And I didn't have to suffer an aesthetic imbalance, either, because Rosemary had trotted me right out to get a new bra with a perky silicone bosom that slipped into the right pocket, perfectly matching my left breast. Thank God for Nordstrom's.

Ole was spending so much time caregiving and driving me he couldn't meet his bow orders. A violinist from the Boston Symphony Orchestra wanted a second bow to go with the one Ole had made him several years before, and the cellist from the Emerson String Quartet was eager to try one of Ole's magic wands. So Rosemary's pilot friend Dave offered to ferry me to the Font—and back to the Peninsula—which would save Ole six hours of driving time. When I climbed into that twin-engine plane and Dave accelerated down the runway, my spirits lifted with the wings. I felt like the piece of tangerine-pink fabric Sas had sent me ("I thought you could use some color!"). I was that swag of shimmery silk.

Up in the sky I left all the fear and drama behind. We flew over the Peninsula and where Ole had flown me that day we were headed to hike Mt. Townsend. We skirted Whidbey Island, the shadow of Dave's plane following us to Boeing Field. One afternoon Ole came along, too, and Dave offered him the controls. Ole noted the weather and dipped us down below the heavy cloud cover to find our way home. "Scud-running!" he said.

Scud-running was Ole's and my modus operandi. One morning Badger jumped on the bed as usual to wake us up, and Ole said, "What's this?" as our mustachioed cat pushed his head into Ole's hand for a stroke. I reached over and felt it, too: a lump on Badger's shoulder. "Noooooooo…," I said, yet another rush of panic obliterating any brain function. We took him to the vet right away—me in my buff and pale, puffy face—and I wept when the vet told us Badger had a tumor. He'd have to undergo surgery right away. "He's an old cat, almost 20," the vet said. "I'm a little concerned about his getting through the anesthetic. I'd say there's a fifty-fifty chance he'll make it. But if he does, we've bought him some time." The earliest he could schedule surgery was on my Font Day the following week.

In the meantime, I went to see that horse. When I got to the meadow, Buddy was grumpy and laid his ears back. When I tried to lunge him on the end of the lead rope, he tossed his head in excitement, then trotted right by me, nipping my arm on the way. I jumped back, shocked and horrified by this terrible blow to my connection. Had I misread him? Done things wrong? Had the carrots in my pocket made him nippy? I sank to an all-time low. The bruise where he'd bitten me swelled up a bit, but I didn't tell Ole. Dr. Allie had told me to be extra careful. But Buddy needed work! I wished desperately I knew someone in town who could help me. I googled "nipping in horses," but nothing satisfactory popped up. I went to bed with Badger, who was completely unbothered about any ideas of surgery or a nippy horse. He snoozed and purred.

A friend of Rosemary's had heard that I was befriending a horse in the middle of treatment, and she loaned me a set of DVDs that featured a husband-wife team who developed seven games to get to know your horse. It was something I hadn't thought of, and I eagerly opened up the package. They were interesting, but nothing like the Bedouin on YouTube. Plus, my brain just didn't seem to accommodate anything remotely connected to instruction. After the nipping incident, I couldn't even think of "training" anymore. I just wanted to be with Buddy. After writing my friend Peggy in Boston about how he had hurt my feelings and had nipped me while frisking around, she wrote, *"Chances are that most of Buddy's unhelpful behavior was, at one time, exactly the thing that enabled him to get through…with his spirit and self intact."*

Peggy's take on Buddy made me realize that I just needed to hang out with that horse and not try to tackle things I wasn't sure of, especially when my strength was not exactly at its peak. I remembered when I sat down under the tree, Buddy had picked up a stick and thrown it up in the air, and it landed near his feet. He'd picked it up again and brought it over, dropping it right in front of me. I always seemed to laugh aloud when I was with him.

Peggy's second email on the subject of Buddy:

> *That night in the garden of Gethsemane has always struck me deeply—Jesus just wanted someone to stay awake and BE with him during that long, dark night. Certainly, there is a time for fixing and therapy and working-with. But even then, getting too caught up in the doing and fixing…can be counter-productive…*

I remembered the round marble Peggy had given me the afternoon after we had lunch with her father. Inside the deep blue swirly a cloud of white shone like a horse's mane.

> *Now to be specific to Buddy, it sure sounds as though you both are on the same page of life—what you can give right now, and receive right now, sounds to me exactly suited to what he can give and receive right now. It sounds just perfect to just BE with him.…Sometimes you just need to know someone is there.*

That night, the Purification kicked in with full force, and Haas came to me in a dream. His face lit up when he saw me because we were giving a party. We discussed the menu—his famous Lebanese yogurt soup, and a lemon chicken—when all of a sudden he said, "I have to go."

"What?" I said in a panic, reaching out to him. "Where are you going!?" His face went soft, his extraordinary dark-lashed eyes warm with purpose. "Not to worry," he said, his figure fading, "I've just got something to take care of."

I woke with a start, and the full, orangey moon shone through a layer of late-summer mist, rendering the night prehistoric and otherworldly. Ole rocked me back and forth, back and forth, rubbing my back while I whimpered with the new effects of the Font. I clicked the CD player poised with Gregorian chants, and they glided quietly through the night like guardians. Across the Straits toward the back side of Whidbey Island, the old, familiar foghorn sighed. I fought with an existential fear. Was I dying? Was Badger dying, too? Why was I losing things right and left? Was there any way out?—until finally I surrendered, letting the questions wash over me without demanding an answer.

Then we heard a strange noise, a primitive call so old it could have been Yahweh Himself. I turned my head on the pillow so both ears could catch the strange caw as it flew within a foot of our open window. In the moonlight the outline of a great blue heron pumped its huge pterodactyl wings toward the lagoon near the beach. Out of the void a bird's voice braided Ole and me to the deep, timeless rhythms of the Earth, right in the middle of my own creature-crisis. The heron, like the tree frog, helped me accept the unknowing, to embrace what it means to be here or not here. I was discovering that both are viable states. I wore these new-found feelings like raiment. I was seeing myself from a *where* I had not known before, a Land of Time Bending. My body was matter bending to light.

Every time I arrived for my appointment with Dr. Allie before the infusion, I'd made it a habit to bring her a poem in a sealed envelope. The day of Badger's surgery, however, I brought nothing except my tears. I told her my cat was in surgery right at that moment. Dr. Allie, the smallest doctor on the planet, picked up a box of Kleenex, brought it to me sitting on the exam table, pulled one out, and offered it like a flower.

When I got to the Font, Kris said that she was praying for Badger. In fact, word had got out, and apparently the whole oncology unit seemed to be praying that my cat would make it through surgery that day. Jen, Patrick, Lisa at the front desk, the whole crowd. When the familiar whiff of saline solution flushed through the chemo port, I also knew I was heading back to the Underworld again. "It's a little bumpy right now," I told Kris.

She laid her soft hand on mine. "I know," she said.

That night back at Rosemary's, Freddie served us up some beef stew. Mine remained untouched. When the phone rang, Celia jumped up to get the phone, "I'll bet it's Ooooooooola!!!! I'll bet he's calling about His Badgesty!" My heart stepped up.

"Hi Ole!" Celia's little voice chirped into the phone. "Okay... here she is."

My hand shook as I picked up the phone. But there was my husband's voice, the sound of normalcy.

"Badger's made it through. He's home," Ole said. "He's purring right now. Can you hear him? Here—I'll put him on speaker phone." My face said it all. Rosemary's hands waved and Freddie smiled. I punched the speaker button on Rosemary's phone. A huge purr filled Rosemary's living room.

"The Badgepipe!! The Badgepipe!!" Celia said, skipping around the living room.

"Same old Badger," Ole said. "I'll sleep on the floor with him tonight, to help him get to the litter box. We're going to get some more use out of this old cat yet."

Chapter 40.

Rays of Illumination

DURING MY TIME IN RIOJOS, one of its most notable residents was the reclusive abstract painter Agnes Martin. The year before I left town, she surprised the local art museum with a gift of several of her paintings. The creamy, blue-and-white, horizontal-lined paintings hung in a softly lit room in a temple-like hush. Before the opening, I was asked to interview her in her small apartment, not far from Riojos Plaza. We sat at her kitchen table, her level gaze as unencumbered as the smooth graphite lines across her canvases. At eighty-five, she wore a cheerful smock that matched the blue of the New Mexico sky, striped socks, and red sneakers. "I feel happy when I keep looking at a painting and I can imagine it completed," Agnes Martin told me. "Before I start a painting, I have a complete inspiration in my mind…" She engaged with something outside the window I could not see. "When you're in this rat race, you need to turn your back to the world and rest. It's so quiet, looking out…"

Agnes Martin's words came back to me in mid-January when I embarked on the final phase of the BCA—two full months of daily radiation. Dr. Hunter had arranged for my treatment on the Peninsula so I wouldn't have to make the long drive to Seattle, and Ole made a schedule. Friends and volunteers drove me an hour each way to what I called "The Rays of Illumination," where Agnes Martin's "quiet" was palpable.

Each morning I was transported around the bay shrouded with Douglas firs, branches hanging like sodden sleeves. And when we emerged out into the alluvial plain where sea and mountains meet, Martin's words rose to the surface: "People tell me my paintings are about peace," she said. "But really, I think they're about tranquility. Tranquility comes when you are resting."

On those daily drives I, too, was looking out from a place removed. I remembered a night years before, when Celia, Rosemary, and I had stood outside my beach cottage in the middle of the night, dazzled by the emerald radiance of the Northern Lights. Celia, barely four at the time, gazed at the heavens and said, "Ohhhhhhhhhhhh!" her upheld fists clenched in delight, "I've waited my *whole life* to see the Northern Lights!!"

I wondered if I'd waited my whole life to feel what I was feeling in this Breast Cancer Adventure, even in the throes of physical discomfort: a shimmering inside me that I might only describe as tenderness—for my precious body, for the people, the animals and the aliveness of this world. My body felt like it was reaching out, contracting and expanding into the dome of the sky. Was there a difference? Was this what they called the Holy Spirit?

And while I offered up my body to that giant machine and welcomed the horizontal bands of light fixed on the canvas of my torso, I embraced the notion that those rays were also scorching out any residue in my character that needed scrubbing. Each time Juliet, my technician, placed me on the cold metallic table, she covered me in blankets, so I would be warm and still during the zapping.

"The response to art should be emotion," Martin had told me, her strong, wrinkled hands folded quietly on the table. "Everybody's making the mistake of thinking they have to *understand* art, that it's intellectual. But no. I think that people don't pay enough attention to their feelings." She handed me the Gold Lion Award she'd won at the Venice Biennale the year before, a coveted prize for all artists. I hefted the small, heavy treasure. She said she liked the Lion, but she was more interested in what her *paintings* were getting at.

"I don't mind that people think my paintings are landscapes," she set the Lion back on the windowsill. Outside the sky looked like an azure pool. "I like to think they are a far view. I think human beings are capable of responding *beyond* the world."

It wasn't until I experienced these rituals of healing—The Font, The Purification Rites, and the Rays of Illumination—that Martin's words spoke to me with more depth. As I had succumbed first to the death of my parents, to Haas, to the news of cancer, then to the surgery, followed by the Underworld of chemotherapy, and finally radiation, I'd moved into an odd calm, as if I were watching myself, just going along for the ride. In my yoga practice Noelle would say, "Who is observing all these feelings come and go? Who is that Quiet inside of you when your body is in pain? Who is sitting in the audience watching the other 'you' on stage, fractured with fear?"

This calm dovetailed with my growing relationship with Buddy, especially on the days I just sat in the meadow with him and the mules. When I recognized the pocket of quiet inside myself, I noticed that his behavior mirrored mine. And, driving to the Rays of Illumination with my friends (who respected my need for silence), a radiant joy began to pulse through me, a gratitude for things beyond they physical. Those glittering blue-and-white Olympic Mountain snowfields were part of me, my body's abstract landscape.

"Christine, I know you're in the middle of radiation," my friend Cathy said on the phone. "But Abel's school needs a poet. Like now. The poet they booked doesn't *do* little kids."

I'd always considered the many elementary school gigs I'd done for years as fun, but not my *real* work. And I'd been off the grid for nearly a year. Could I face classrooms of children? What about my pale skin? My weird fuzz-head of newly sprouted platinum hair?

"They have to spend this money," Cathy continued, "It's not a bad chunk of change. Can you do it?"

The following week, after Ole took me to the Rays and back, I drove the half mile across town to F Street Elementary. I teetered in with my two flutes and a basket of poems. The children were returning from recess, and the hallway smelled like rain, wet wool, and lunchroom pizza.

"Hey!!! I LOVE your hair!" a little girl said as she hopped past me and waved. I reached up and lay a hand to my head. Who knew it would be fashionable?

When I arrived at Teacher Dawn's kindergarten class, the children were seated in a half circle on the floor. One little girl in a pink dress reached into my basket and patted my flute.

"Ohhhhhhhhh," they said. "Ohhhhhhhhhh."

"Boys and girls, can you say hello to Christine?"

"Hellooooooooooooooooooooooooooooooo!" They wriggled like puppies.

I bent my rickety legs to settle on the miniature chair. "Today I thought we'd sing and make some poems. What do you think of that?"

"Oh, yesssssssssssssssssssssss!" they said. A few clapped their hands.

We sang about the wind and talked about how poems come from dancing. After I played them a jig, Devon said that he could make that exact tune—by whistling. "Well," I said, picking up my flute again. "With a claim like that, we'd better play it together." Devon climbed over his classmates to stand close beside me. His front teeth were missing, but he blew air through his mouth so hard his forehead wrinkled.

We sang another song about turtles in the sun, and I recited a poem about my cat Badger when he was a kitten. I'd written it for Massachusetts schoolchildren in my Boston days when I'd take Badger with me in a basket, his white vest and black mustache a big hit with the children. Once he'd nearly nabbed a fish in the classroom fish tank. Another time he'd dug up a few bean sprouts. The kids loved him, and his mustache was always a big hit. I showed these kindergartners a drawing I'd made of Badger and then clapped with them:

> Badger in the saucepan
> Badger on the stair.
> Badger in the looking glass,
> Badger in my hair…

They screamed with laughter.

"I have a cat!" Anika said.

"I have TWO cats," Lizzy stood up.

"My uncle's cat died," Devon said quietly.

"That must have been sad," I said.

"Yes, it was." More wrinkles in the brow. "We buried him near the sandbox." I did not tell Devon that Badger himself was dying as we spoke. He'd bounced back after the surgery, but a few months later he began to sleep more and breathe less deeply. Ole and I had fixed up a nice nest for him on the heated bathroom floor, but soon I knew he'd be joining Devon's uncle's cat.

I passed out little scraps of colored paper. Each of us crayoned a picture that showed how we were feeling at that moment. One kid drew a sun, another made jiggly lines, another a black spot. Devon drew an X. Soon we had a long line of tiny pictures across the floor. A picture-poem stretched out like a horizon.

Before leaving, I played them a final tune on my flute. I'd not played much at all during my illness. What came out, however, seemed to originate from a new place. I wasn't really making the notes at all; they were making me. I closed my eyes, and Devon laid a tiny hand on my knee. I felt the others squinching closer.

When I finished, I opened my eyes and the room was completely silent. Suddenly, they all scrambled up and, like Velcro, attached themselves to me anywhere they could—my legs, arms, waist, even my basket.

"Don't go!" they cried. "Don't goooo!" I had to sit right back down in the tiny chair, fighting tears. I wrapped my arms around as many little bodies as I possibly could. My eyelashes had yet to come back, so I still couldn't blink properly. But the tears helped, and when I dug a Kleenex out of my pocket and wiped my eyes, all I could see was a sea of children washing over me, swirling with the last words Agnes Martin had said to me long ago: "Did you ever get up in the morning and feel happy without cause?"

Chapter 41.

⟿ *Winds of Heaven* ⟾

AFTER MY FINAL DOSE OF radiation, a friend invited me to work part-time at the local organic vegetable farm. When I hesitated, she said, "Come on—it'll help you get back in the swing of things." I reluctantly agreed, even though I pictured a passel of hippie wannabees with bumper stickers that said: I FARM YOU EAT. But the workers, ranging in age from twenty to seventy, were friendly and without affectation, including a young barista, a retired real estate agent, and a recent college graduate who was opening his own brewery with beer made from Douglas fir trees.

By June we were all eating our lunch outside instead of in the greenhouse. Seven of us sat at a picnic table and passed around fresh spinach salad and lentil soup. I shed my sweatshirt in the warm June sun. In the weeks of weeding and planting, I hadn't said a word about my cancer treatment (nor that my own healing brew—Taxol—originated in the sap of a Northwest yew tree), but as the season unfolded I had told them about this horse Buddy I was spending time with. It seemed like safe lunchtime conversation.

"The trouble is, it's like being involved with a married man," I told my fellow vegetable farmers.

"A married man?!" they laughed nervously, shaking their heads.

"What do you mean?" Barbara, a fiftyish woman with a big smile, helped herself to more salad. "Are you having an *affair* with Buddy?" Everyone laughed.

"Well, you're not far off," I said, flexing my aching fingers, still stiff and sore from treatment. "Buddy is owned by my neighbor. And now that I'm starting to ride him more, I want to make sure I'm not overstepping with Fred. Even though he's cool with me spending so much time with Buddy…I just don't know…" I was conscious of figuring this out as I was telling the story. "So for the last week or so I've just stayed away from him…" They all looked up.

"Stayed away from him?" Barbara put down her fork.

The truth was, I wasn't concerned about Fred—he was delighted with my spending time with Buddy. After all, I only rode him around in the Bluff Meadow field. And I wasn't really troubled that Fred owned him; I had no idea how Ole and I could ever afford a horse. The problem was that the more I was with Buddy, the more attached I became. And the more attached I became, the possibility of losing him loomed larger (would Fred decide to sell him? Or ask someone else to ride him, too?). Right now I was at a tipping point, that place in any relationship where you can still get out without too much collateral damage to the heart. I was finished with treatment; I was getting healthier and stronger every day. And, after more than a year, I was getting my life back. (As if such a thing were possible: do we ever get our old lives "back," after death or illness?) Now would be the time to unhitch myself.

Sebastian, the tanned farm manager, passed me some fresh bread baked by his wife, Kelly. "Well, why don't you ride Buddy up here? We can all meet him. And hey, we can put him in the field while you're working." He gently tucked a stray black strand of hair behind his ear, then pointed to the large fenced field abutting both the forest and the acres of raspberries, strawberries, and green vegetables, some already peeking through the ground. "I'll even fix the fence for you!"

"You mean—? I could ride him up *here?*"

In a rush of nervous excitement, I suddenly viewed a new wide-angled picture coming into focus: Buddy and me with a real destination. A reason to ride. An adventure all our own. Of course, the farm seemed a continent away from Bluff Meadow (how would I get here exactly?), but with Sebastian's invitation came an instant expansion of what was possible, as if the Known World had suddenly enlarged to encompass vast regions of wildness and delight. All thoughts of unhitching myself from Buddy vanished into the June marine air.

"You're going to ride Buddy out of the big field?" Ole looked up from his laptop where he was cruising the Paragliding Forum again. Though he'd quit flying during my treatment, he was eager to launch his wing again. Paddleboarding was fun, "but nothing beats the air," he'd said.

"Yes, well, I asked Fred, and he was surprised that I hadn't done that yet already." I sat down next to Ole on the couch.

"You haven't really ridden him much at all," he said. "Are you feeling up to it? Buddy's not exactly a calm horse from what you've told me. Good for sitting *beside*, but riding *on top of*?"

I hadn't told him that I'd been riding Buddy more and more with just a halter in the big field.

"Fred said Buddy needs work," I said, "that his intelligence and energy need focusing. I think I'm going to ride Buddy up to Frog Hill. Maybe not while I'm working" (I knew I'd be too preoccupied with him to pick strawberries), "but Friday is the day we pick up our own vegetables...I was thinking maybe I'd wear a backpack and..."

Ole took a short breath. He'd seen Buddy snorting and racing around like a wildman in that field with the mules. In a nano-second, however, my husband's navigational passions overrode his reservations. "Let's get on Google Earth and see what trails you would take to get there. In fact, if I remember from riding my bike through that forest years ago, you can get to Frog Hill from Buddy's meadow…hmmm…except for that short stretch of Henry Street…without hitting any roads." My heart leapt.

The following Friday, with Ole's orientation in my head, I bridled Buddy with one of Lightfoot's bridles I'd found in a box of my childhood treasures and softened up with olive oil. I led him out the gate, sidled him up to a sawhorse, and slipped on his bare back. Fred hadn't offered his saddle, and I couldn't imagine buying one with all the stacked-up medical bills. The empty pack on my back rustled, and Buddy jumped sideways a couple feet. I pressed my red Gortex REI hat more firmly on my head. My heart picked up its pace. I nudged Buddy toward the gate and out we went, pointing south toward Copp's Wood, Buddy's head high. The June sunshine made every dewy leaf glint; the smell of low tide wafted up the bluff.

Buddy and I were headed into unknown territory. I didn't know how he'd behave with cars or how much he'd spook. The backpack moment was enough of a hint, but I didn't feel one ounce of fear. Riding a sparky Arabian on an unknown trail? Without a saddle or a helmet? It didn't even occur to me that this might be foolish. I'd already been through the Valley of the Shadow of Death. What was there to be afraid of now? And, after my last appointment with Dr. Allie, hadn't she said, "Your tests are clean. Now. Go live your life!"

Buddy and I crossed L Street, found the trail into Copp's Wood, and headed into the shadows of the trees. Buddy pranced through the forest as if he, too, were up for a bushwhack. The morning sun shone through the cedars, particles whirling in the cones of light. Bands of sun lay across the trail, and the woods smelled like skunk cabbage and balsam. Buddy seemed to know the way. I stroked his neck and held his reins tight because I knew at any moment he might leap sideways. Wild rhododendrons bloomed in splashes of pink and white among the mossy fir trunks, and the Swainson's thrush called his familiar ascending song.

Awash in gratitude, I was being carried through the fir-needled forest by Buddy's spirit. At one juncture I wondered if we were on the right path, but then I remembered Ole's map and sure enough it looked as if we'd almost reached the southernmost edge of Copp's Wood. I urged Buddy into a canter, and we flew over a huge fallen log. Salmonberries, blackberries, and ocean spray whooshed past my legs.

We emerged from the trees and discovered the driveway to Frog Hill. I slipped off at the gate, unlatched it, and walked him up the long hill to the farm. No one seemed to be around, but there was a greenhouse filled with produce and a list of how much each of us was to take. I managed to stuff my pack full, all while managing Buddy's nonstop fidgeting. The asparagus, chard, and spinach scooshed around on my back as I led Buddy to a stump. I'd had to stuff the beets in at the end, and the pack was top-heavy. Buddy tossed his head and I quickly jumped on, the pack swaying. I hung on and pointed him down the long drive toward the forest where a car happened to be coming in and held the gate for us. By the time we'd found the trail back home, I felt an over-whelming sense of victory. Buddy and I had a purpose! Buddy's back was life itself.

Emerging from the cocoon of cancer treatment (or any trauma, I imagine), the world looks more distinct and shimmery. Dinners I made with the summer vegetables tasted exotic. Ole's face appeared handsome as a Nordic god's. My own body, lean and taut with the muscles I'd built while riding Buddy, felt (almost) like a teenager's. Everything seemed like a celebration. Gary, my astronomer friend, wrote me with exciting news:

*SWAS and your poem are still coursing through the heavens.
Your poem has now traveled more than 1.7 billion miles—or
about 19 times the distance between the Earth and the Sun....
This poem gets around.*

I couldn't help but be proud of it, galloping all that way through dark space. Gary ended with *"The observatory with a poem for its heart is teaching us how stars are born."*

That summer, like one of those endless childhood summers, seemed like a rebirth. The sunny rides in Copp's Wood atop Buddy's warm flat back were like living in a Technicolor movie. Even Badger's death—he chose to leave the day after my very last cancer treatment—was a kind of opening, a window into a life not colored by illness or sadness. He'd given me the gift of hanging on till the very end, and, just shy of his twentieth birthday, he jumped over the mossy log to the other side.

Buddy marched full force into my waking (and dreaming) life. When I rode him to pick up vegetables on Fridays, I found many other trails in town, too. Sometimes I even brought Buddy to our courtyard to visit, which was a protected place for him to graze. I asked Ole if we could stop at the tack shop one day to find a new chinstrap for my bridle. I hadn't been in a tack shop in decades. The leather smell hit me like opening a long-closed cedar chest.

Somehow, I had to find some container for my gratitude. A vessel, a wheelbarrow, or a water bucket to hold my joy. In a million years I couldn't have guessed that I'd be involved with a horse again. And there was so much I wanted to learn.

Which brings us to that day at the end of the vegetable harvest summer. There was a horse trainer, my friend Stephanie said, who was offering a clinic at the Fairgrounds. And his name was Ken. That first lesson with Buddy and Ken remains one of those rare episodes when you know *at that moment* your life has changed. Something shifts.

In the course of one Saturday a new, mysterious world had opened up, and I was just about as excited as Buddy when he dashed across the meadow with Molly and Gracie. What Ken did with Buddy that day resonated with things I'd seen and read when I was laid up in bed for months. Like the Bedouin's in the YouTube video, Ken's commands had been barely visible.

At the end of that First Lesson Day, one of the women offered to let me borrow a saddle she had for sale. It didn't have a girth, and I couldn't ride it home, so Ken said, "I'll be happy to run it down there for you. Where do you live?" I was floored. My newfound teacher offering to deliver a borrowed saddle? I was as nervous as when Mom and I had visited Donald Hall.

"Uh, just down the road," I said.

"I'll catch up with you," Ken said, and I pointed Buddy toward home, hurrying to get there before Ken. (What would Ole say? What on Earth would they say to each other?) When I opened our little courtyard gate, Ken pulled up. I welcomed him, and Ole stepped out the French door. They shook hands, and Ole asked how the training went.

"Great!" I said, turning to look at this man with a cigarette. How would I ever explain to Ole the magic that had happened with Buddy, that wild ripping around the arena, then Ken bringing Buddy back to him with only a motion of his hand?

"Great little setup you have here," Ken said, taking in our house, my little red studio, Ole's shop, and the courtyard.

"Well, we just moved in a year or so ago," Ole said. "We still have a lot of work to do." Meanwhile I held on to Buddy's reins while he chewed on the grass. The men didn't have any problem talking about the structure of the house, drain spouts, and what the weather did to cedar. My mind was on one thing only:

I wanted to go with Buddy to the place Ken had shown me that afternoon.

"Buddy *is* your horse," Anne said, "even if you don't 'own' him." She offered me a fresh scone. Anne was most emphatically not a horse person. "My garden is my horse," she often told me. The birches were beginning to turn yellow, and her exotic beds—she knew all the plants' Latin names—were beautiful even as their leaves faded. Her pines, pruned like huge bonsai trees, were sculptures themselves. Through her studio window, I could see new clay forms taking shape on the wall and on her bench. The yet-unglazed and unpainted shapes—some of them twisting and others looking like big horns and mouths on the wall—were almost alive. They reminded me of Buddy's graceful lines.

"Yes, he is, but that's not it," I said. "It's just that it's hard to share him now." I was bereft. Fred had gone on another pack trip for the weekend, but this time he'd taken the mules and Buddy.

"But you have the horse and you don't have all the bills! And Fred knows how much you love Buddy," Anne said, pouring me another cup of tea.

Anne was right. But it wasn't about "owning." It was still about the fear of Buddy suddenly disappearing, irrational as that sounded. So many loves had disappeared so fast. I didn't want to risk another. And truly, the stronger my body became, the more I wanted to be with my sprightly pal. All through that healing summer and into the fall, when vegetables burgeoned at Frog Hill and the bounty in my life grew bigger than fresh corn, onions, and garlic, I knew there was something more than physical healing going on in my body. Buddy had carried me there. I'd been attending the local Episcopal Church, and one Sunday there was an announcement that the St. Francis Day Animal Blessing was to occur at 3:00 p.m.

That afternoon, Buddy and I navigated the two-and-a-half miles to town, making our way through new trails and quiet streets to the little church overlooking the bay. I rode him right up the sidewalk that abutted the labyrinth and slipped off his back. A wave of "Ohhhhhhhhhh! A horse!!" rippled through the dog and cat owners leaning over their charges. A rabbit sat stock-still in a cardboard box. Three chickens clucked in a cage. A black Lab wore a red scarf, and a tiny bronze poodle curled in a man's lap. I had a sudden flash of when I was a child and Mom had told us: "If there is ever a war or an earthquake and if our family should get separated, go to the nearest Episcopal church, the one with the red wooden door. That's where we'll meet," she said. "No matter what." I had pictured rounding up my hens and cats, our dog Captain following, me swinging Max in his birdcage—a kind of parade to the church with a red door.

"Welcome everyone!" the priest said, holding up her arms, her robe spangled with a hand-sewn chasuble, her spiked gray hair shiny in the October sun. I smoothed Buddy's mane. I was handed a program that Buddy immediately grabbed in his teeth, and the congregation laughed. Buddy nodded his head up and down, the program flapping.

"Turn to the first page and we'll sing together," the priest said, and we all launched into:

> *All things bright and beautiful*
> *All creatures great and small*
> *All things wise and wonderful*
> *The Lord God made them all...*

By the time we reached the end of this hymn my mother had sung to Rosemary, Paul, and me, my face was wet with tears. But Buddy stood happily unmoved, as if he were exactly where he was meant to be. No fidgeting, no jumping around.

Children whispered to their cats, dogs thumped their tails. When it came time for the blessing, the priest used a moistened branch of rosemary to touch each and every animal with care, gently calling them by name.

She dipped the rosemary into the ceramic bowl and, with a quiet knowing, walked toward Buddy and me. "And now—" she smiled and held out her hand gently, "What's this marvelous horse's name?"

"Buddy!" I said, as if he were my firstborn.

Buddy nodded and wrapped his lips around the rosemary branch, its smell prompting him to curl his lips back into a horse-laugh. More chuckles from my fellow pilgrims.

"Ohhhhhhhhhhh, Buddy," the priest said softly, touching his forehead with her palm. "What a wonderful face you have." Buddy nodded while a dog huffed around his legs. A child raced after a puppy. But Buddy did not flinch, nor did he raise his head or puff his nostrils. His eyes remained soft, his hoofs planted firmly on the ground.

The priest raised the branch and touched Buddy's delicate head, tiny beads of water clinging to his forelock like jewels. "In the name of the Creator, the Redeemer, and the Sanctifier, Buddy, I bless you…and oh, what a blessèd soul you are…"

By November, Buddy was a fixture in Ole's and my life. I brought him to our house. He liked to peek in the French doors, too, and one day he stepped right into the dining room. At first Ole was a bit nervous around Buddy (he'd had very little experience with horses), but he was charmed by him, especially when he would accept a carrot through the window or just walk right up to say hello. I came home from riding one day, and Ole presented Buddy and me with a red-and-white halter and lead rope he'd made from a pattern he'd found online. When we put it on Buddy, he looked just like a candy cane. Buddy nibbled on the rosebush, until he heard Fred's diesel truck drive by. His ears perked up, and he whinnied and trotted to the gate. I was jealous, even though I knew Buddy associated Fred's truck with feeding time. Ole quickly went inside and got the camera, hurried around to the front yard, and clicked several pictures of Buddy's cute face in his new, dapper halter, his head just high enough to look over the gate, delicate ears perked toward the next interesting moment.

"I can't stand it," Ole said. "He's so cute. Even when he gives me a grumpy face." I laughed as Buddy stuck his nose out at Ole. Ole held out his hand to Buddy and tickled the whiskers on his chin. My husband was becoming as smitten as I was. And he championed my lessons with Ken. But I had to be realistic: even if Fred were still willing to sell Buddy to us, we had no money. Period. Paragraph.

An aunt had died during the BCA and had left us a small nest egg, but after chipping away at the medical bills, we'd eaten up a good deal of it. Even with medical insurance and Ole selling Kanestrom bows to musicians around the world, we never seemed to catch up. We were still paying for my year of treatment and the follow-up visits stacked up on top of them. The Hempstroms, as we called ourselves, were not exactly flush.

So, the week before Thanksgiving, I agreed to teach a course called "Dealing with Difficult People" at the Department of Energy, over three hundred miles away in Eastern Washington. It was a three-day course I'd tailored for technical people in charge of the Hanford nuclear waste cleanup. I hadn't driven any distance in over a year; it was daunting to think of the snowy mountain pass, the Interstate, and its lonely funnel of traffic across the state. I was surprised at how much I'd depended on Ole's driving during the previous year and surprised at myself for approaching the job with trepidation. But Ole reminded me how I'd taught another three-day class, "Giving the Winning Presentation," at the US Navy right after the Font of Purification, the week before I'd started radiation. It had been one of my most successful courses, primarily because I wasn't thinking about how I should "professionally come across." The first day of that course I'd told the participants that my headgear was not a fashion statement, but that I'd just finished chemotherapy for cancer. The room fell silent, but I then told them that this, for me, was the perfect example of giving a presentation. Each time we prepare for presenting, we plan *what* we want to say, but there are always conditions we cannot predict: a headache, a difficult colleague in the conference room, a fight with a spouse that morning. Or chemotherapy. When we acknowledge these things (if only to ourselves), we can actually be more present for the people in the room, and teach or speak to *them*, not just the subject matter. After three days, those officers, civilians, and enlisted Navy employees gave stirring presentations, including on topics sometimes fraught such as shipboard gender issues.

Now I was seven months out of treatment, and the elation I'd felt all summer could be channeled back into work. I packed my suitcase for the D.O.E. and headed out over those snowy mountains, gaining confidence all over again, in things as simple as driving. I marveled at the mind's ability to bounce back along with the body.

Before I'd left for Eastern Washington, Ole had mentioned that he might just *ask* Fred about Buddy, about how much he might cost if we were the buy him. My heart expanded with such a possibility, but even if Fred agreed to sell us Buddy for cheap, Ole had no idea how expensive horses were. It wasn't the cost of the horse exactly—it was everything from farriers to salt licks. Still, to think that Ole was actually entertaining the idea of Buddy being ours—it took my breath away, even when I knew Buddy already "had" me. In fact, he had Ole, too.

I arrived back home the day before Thanksgiving, tired but happy. I'd barely gotten in the door and hugged my husband hard, when Ole said, "So I had a talk with Fred."

I dropped my bags with a thump.

Ole took two beers out of the fridge and opened them both, handing me one and sinking into a kitchen chair. I sat down too, my hands shaking.

"What did he say?" A surge of unbridled hope coursed through me, as if the list of Rational Reasons Against Horse Ownership had burned up in the fire now crackling in our fireplace. Maybe there was a way around the money problem after all. I couldn't see it, but maybe Ole could.

"Well, it's not what I'd hoped." Ole set his beer on the table. Just as those words left his mouth, I had the sickening thought that Fred—knowing we were broke—might have gone ahead and sold Buddy to someone else. Fred had found Buddy another home. I closed my eyes and squeezed them tight, the dread moving up from my belly and into my chest.

"I asked him about selling Buddy to us…" Ole cleared his throat. "But Fred said he's having second thoughts, and he just wants to keep him." Ole pushed his bottle of beer to the side and folded his hands on the table. "He's so glad that you've had a good year with Buddy—and you can still continue to ride and do everything you're doing now—lessons with Ken—"

In one, clean movement I lurched from the kitchen table directly to the couch, landing face down on the cushions, my body emptied of all energy. A deluge of grief splattered all over the sofa, the living room, my husband, the world at large. It dampened the chandelier, the windows, the memory of all the recent losses, the litany of almost-hads raining down from the ceiling and pooling onto the floor. Callie came up on the sofa and purred by my head.

My outburst took me by surprise as much as it did Ole. Until that moment I didn't know how deeply invested I'd been in the idea of having Buddy as my own. I'd fantasized, yes, but I hadn't fully realized how big a role Buddy played in moving forward with my life.

"Oh, Christine…" Ole sat next to me, his face pained and conflicted.

"It just goes really deep for me, this horse thing…it's not about horses. But *a* horse." I hiccupped with crying.

How could I articulate to Ole the hold a horse can have on you? It can last a lifetime. During a lesson with Ken just the previous week, Buddy had been agitated, and Ken was asking me to help him face his fear. When Ken invited me to get bigger and give Buddy a stronger aid when I was turning him, I'd actually burst into tears, something I'd never ever done in front of Ken.

"I just don't want to let Buddy down," I'd said, bringing Buddy to a halt. Ken looked at me with a huge question mark on his face. I got off Buddy and searched my pocket for a Kleenex.

"He represents life to you, doesn't he?" Ken said. I hadn't really talked about it much, but Ken knew I was fresh out of cancer treatment.

"Yes, but that's not all of it. I feel as if I abandoned Lightfoot. Let him down in some way." Just the thought of my childhood horse brought on another sob. "I never want to do that again." I blew into my Kleenex.

I'd told Ken I'd had a horse in my teens, but I hadn't revealed to him my sorrow until that moment in the wind. I kept to myself all the haunting nightmares I'd had over the years—of finding Lightfoot starving in a stable, of him running to find me in unfamiliar fields, and the sound of his whinny calling me in my subconscious.

"How old did you say Lightfoot was when you sold him?" Ken didn't bat an eye when my nose dripped onto my jacket.

"Twelve," I said, reaching out to Buddy, suddenly aware that Buddy was the same age.

"But, Christine. Lightfoot was the grown-up then. Not you." Ken grabbed the top of his hat to hold it down in the westerly gust. Buddy cocked his hip and relaxed by resting his hind foot. "I imagine Lightfoot understood you had to grow up sometime. We all do. Including our horses. You didn't know it then, but when you left home, you had to let each other go. You thought you were taking care of Lightfoot," Ken blew his cigarette smoke toward the ground. "When really, he was taking care of you."

I hardly felt Ole rise from the couch and fly upstairs. I thought he was getting me an ibuprofen or more Kleenex, but there were sounds of paper being pulled out of the drawer and another measure of quiet. I lay there exhausted—from weeping, from all the miles of driving, from teaching, and all the things I'd never really had in the first place being snatched away.

Ole shot down the stairs in gazelle-like leaps and sat next to me again, this time with a piece of paper in his hand. It was hastily folded into what looked like a greeting card.

"What's this?" I said, sitting up to reach for my glasses.

On the front, in Ole's distinct printing was written:

> The winds of heaven...

I opened up the card.

> ...blow between the ears
> of a horse.
> *Buddy Hempstrom YUP!*

"What?!" I looked up at my husband's face, unable to comprehend this new turn. "Are you kidding?"

"I wanted to surprise you for Christmas—Fred and I concocted a huge, complicated plan to keep this a secret, but oh, it was the wrong thing to do." Ole lifted his arms and dropped them into his lap. "I was going to dress him up on Christmas morning and bring him here to the courtyard. Oh, I'm so so so sorry...you were so upset just now. It's just that—I bought him while you were gone!" he said, grinning. His hair was sticking out every which way. "But this works out fine, doesn't it? Now he's a Thanksgiving present! It saves me having to get a big ribbon to tie around his neck."

"You mean Buddy's—really—?" I sobbed again, this time in utter joy.

"Yes, he's yours now, sweetheart. There's no going back."

Chapter 42.

∽Broken Glass∽

WHEN CHRISTMASTIME DID COME, I bought Buddy a red rubber ball with a handle, wrapped it, and put it under our tree. Ole got a stock heater so Buddy's and the mules' water tub wouldn't freeze over. (Who knew a quiet Norwegian could morph into Nathan Sinclair?) Shortly after that, Ken found us a great deal on a nearly new horse trailer. I sent out Christmas cards with the photo Ole had taken of Buddy peeking over the gate in his candy-cane halter. When I said, one night, that I wished Buddy could be right there in our living room like Bedouin horses in the tents, Ole said, "Wanna go see him?" and we jumped in the car and zipped over to the barn. Buddy's eyes blinked in the dimmed headlights, the mules huffing around the edges. It was like looking into a Christmas crèche. Except, instead of a papier-mâché Baby Jesus there was Buddy, glowing in the night.

The Friday before Christmas, I decorated the house for the family's arrival. Just as I finished hanging stockings for Catharine, Margie, Libby, and Celia, my phone rang. Stephanie wanted to know if I'd join her for a ride on the Barry-Cook Trail, a six-mile, converted railroad grade that curves through the woods and opens out along the south shore of town. Her new horse Willie, a buckskin quarter horse, was proving to be a solid companion for her, and they were doing excellent work with Ken. It was late in the day, but we met halfway and rode at a swift trot side by side on the open track. The horses' breath matched the color of the darkening sky. Our own breath came out in small clouds, and I tightened my wool scarf, glad for my gloves. The cold air and the excitement of riding with another horse made Buddy extra frisky. He lifted his tail high and swished around the long bend in step with Willie. We stopped at a beach overlook and had a snack, letting the horses graze. Though only 3:30 p.m., it was already getting dark, the shortest day of the year. We decided to turn back. Buddy pranced and tossed his head, eager to get home. After leaving the Barry-Cook, the trail narrows in the forest, and Stephanie and I had to ride single-file. I was always extra careful to keep Buddy a good distance from another horse's hindquarters, but as we made a narrow turn Buddy nosed one hoof-fall too close to Willie's tail.

I heard the thud of metal on bone a split second after Buddy lurched left. Before Stephanie even knew what had happened, I'd already swung off Buddy and was kneeling next to his shaking, bloody foreleg. My own legs trembling, I took in the damage. Stephanie was off her horse and with one hand holding Willie's rein, she bent down to examine Buddy's knee. "Damn," she said. "That doesn't look good at all. Oh. I am so sorry, so sorry..." We both knew there was no one to blame. It's what horses do, and sometimes we are on the bad side of luck. She pointed to the smaller—less bloody—but deeper laceration on Buddy's trembling knee. I called Ole and asked him to bring the trailer right away to the turnout nearest the forest trail. Within a half hour, Ole and the trailer had arrived. I was grateful for his driving, as hauling a horse trailer (as we'd had occasion to do for a few faraway training clinics) was stressful for me even in clear daylight. The responsibility of such precious cargo made even the shortest trip a significant undertaking. We loaded both horses, dropped Willie and Stephanie at her barn, and began the hour's trek to the vet.

A small light shone in the parking lot as we pulled into the veterinary hospital. No other trucks or trailers. Ole unclipped the halter tie from the outside of the trailer window, and I carefully backed Buddy out and into the damp, cold night. We heard a high-pitched whinny from inside the building. When the vet opened the giant door, light from the cavernous room made us all blink. Buddy perked his ears and his head went up.

I was disappointed that the on-call vet was not Dr. Claire, Buddy's regular doctor. This woman looked awfully young. But she was all business as she opened the door wider and invited us to the open space where she could inspect Buddy's leg. Buddy was completely obliging, but it was clear he wanted to face the lone horse in the nearby stall, a bay gelding with a perfect white blaze. Closer inspection revealed a ghoulish, three-foot zipper of fresh stitches S-curving all along the horse's flank. He stood utterly still, eyes wide, as if in shock.

"What happened to him?" I asked as the vet kneeled to examine Buddy's wounds.

"It's been all over the news tonight," she paused, as if searching for words. "He was struck by a semi on Route 3." The huge room fell silent except for the hum of the antiseptic lights and the breathing of two horses. Ole touched my hand.

"But Cash is the lucky one. His three pasture mates were killed." She daubed Buddy's knee with gauze soaked in betadine, the iodine color mixing with the red-pink already staining his white leg.

Just the thought of horses running blind down a road is enough to give any horse person nightmares. I'd caught my share of loose ponies—one a pregnant mare from Riojos Pueblo galloping down a main highway at night, a terrifying experience, but I managed to get her off to the side of the road and help the tribal police bring her home. Cash's story was the worst I'd heard. It chilled me to the marrow. Not only that, we later learned that vandals had purposely cut the pasture fence and the horses wandered on the highway at night, panicked by oncoming headlights. Apparently, Cash had been calling out nonstop for his friends since he'd come to the hospital. Until Buddy arrived.

"Well, I don't like the looks of this," the vet said as her slender, expert fingers separated the flaps of skin on the knee wound. A rush of heat and adrenaline coursed through my limbs and I felt dizzy. "What do you mean?" I said, one hand on Buddy's lead rope, the other reaching for my husband's arm.

"Well, with a wound like this—" she curled a long wisp of blonde hair behind her ear and pointed to the vertical cut above the knee. "It's not a big deal, even though it looks worse. We can stitch this up easily. But here—" she squeezed around the small gash on the knee, "the blow may have punctured the synovial joint sac. If that's the case…it's…" she cleared her throat, "potentially very serious." She lifted her finger to show us the liquid that had come out of the wound. "See? If this is synovial fluid, it should be more viscous. It might already be infected. If so, it's a tricky business."

"You mean it couldn't heal? But he's not even lame." My voice became thin like a piece of straw. "Are you saying we'd have to put him down?" I began to shake.

"Well, it's just super hard to heal if it's inside the joint." She stood up and wiped her hands with an antiseptic towel. "I've worked with a lot of racehorses and this is something that happens a lot…but we don't know yet about this injury." She turned toward the medical cabinets against the wall. "First we have to take an X-ray to make sure there are no bone shards in there as well."

Ole put his arm around me and the room began to wobble. Suddenly the bay horse's nightmare and my own were tethered together.

Buddy, who was usually inquisitive and busy, calmly lifted his foreleg for the X-ray block. From a few feet away, Cash watched us intently, keeping Buddy in his sights.

"Cash sure has quieted down since Buddy got here," the vet said as she held the digital plate next to Buddy's knee. I lay my hand on Buddy's neck to keep him quiet and still. He'd helped me quiet me down when I'd staggered through X-rays, MRIs, and myriad tests. Just knowing he was in the world had slowed my racing pulse, and his friendship cheered me on through subsequent months of treatment.

"Okay," the vet said, leaning in to look carefully at the images. "No breaks." She betrayed a small smile and turned the computer screen so we could see. "So now the best thing is to pump him with antibiotics and get a head start on anything that might be happening in there." While she gathered syringes, I pressed my nose to Buddy's neck, inhaling his delicious smell.

The evening unfolded in a blur while she stitched wounds, gave Buddy a sedative, applied a tourniquet, and injected antibiotics directly into the whole knee area as well as into the joint itself. "We'll know tomorrow when I get the white blood cell count in Buddy's knee," she said. "And we can also insert some dye when we take another X-ray to see if the sac is compromised. We'll watch for swelling, too. He'll have to stay for at least one night. The stalls in the outdoor barn are for horses without intravenous medication."

My heart sank. Outside alone? I remembered his weaving at the Fairgrounds. I couldn't imagine him out there in the night by himself. It made me think of my hospital room immediately after cancer surgery when my heart had unexpectedly flipped into atrial fibrillation. I'd been rushed to the ICU and hooked up to scary tubes and humming wires, trapped in pain and discomfort. Ole and Rosemary couldn't come in; the Critical Care Unit didn't allow visitors. I had been alone.

Except for Stephen, the night nurse. He not only fetched a cool fan for my bedside, he also provided me psychic comfort. At a particularly dark moment, I asked if he'd mind holding my hand for a second or two. Without hesitation he reached over the bed bars and clasped it with just the right amount of pressure. Not too tight, but firm enough to transmit a strong dose of empathy. Stephen repeated that wordless act of kindness on and off through the long night.

Cash offered a quiet nicker across the room. His intelligent eyes took in our every move. Cash, I thought. Cash would be here.

"Excuse me," I said to the vet as she wrapped Buddy's leg in thick bandages. "But Buddy doesn't really like to be alone. Would it be possible for him to stay the night in here? With Cash?"

She glanced at Cash whose eyes were fixed on Buddy, and Buddy on him.

"Well, sure. Sure, of course. I don't see why not, it's empty anyway. Here. Put him in the one next to Cash." I led Buddy into the stall with a thick bedding of fresh pine-shavings. Buddy immediately went to the screened window where he could see Cash.

"I won't be here tomorrow till late morning," the vet said, pulling on her down vest, "but we should have the results by the afternoon." As Ole and I left the hospital, the horses' noses were still pressed to the screen, quietly whispering things only horses know. Driving home in the dark, all I could fix my mind on were two very familiar words: "Test results."

That night I didn't sleep at all. Somewhere in the murky region between night and dawn, I reached over to inhale the smell of Ole's smooth shoulder, reassuring myself he was still there. And then I remembered Miss Love, my second-grade teacher. I simply loved Miss Love. The way she smelled. The way she embodied her name and had an uncanny way of knowing who each of us really was, very much like my own mother. She praised my drawings and my stories, and I reveled in her spelling lists. Each weekly set of words felt like a family that fit together. "Coat, Paint, Clean." I loved how the vowel sounds could change everything. "Coat, Paint, Clean."

Miss Love pronounced them like she was family with the words, too. Like she knew how they marched across the page with their own musical step.

But one day she told us that she was getting married and moving to Seattle. I nearly fell out of my desk chair. I came home and told my mother the terrible news and collapsed into a big cry. Mom, in her snip-snap way, suggested that during school vacation, we could have her over to lunch. It was the perfect antidote. Mom laid out the best silver and linen napkins for the chicken salad. There were fresh yellow roses on the table. I was breathless: Miss Love was actually in my own house. We all laughed a lot, especially when our big, white dog Captain flopped down right on Miss Love's feet. When we were having cake, however, Miss Love mentioned that her name would change, too, after the wedding. I stopped eating. I had barely adjusted to her leaving, but leaving her name, too? How would she be Miss Love if she weren't Miss Love? How would she know who she was if she changed her name? After she'd gone, I expressed this new worry to Mom. She told me that Miss Love would always be Miss Love. "But sometimes you lose things," she said. "Even if it's only a name." She began clearing the table, where Miss Love's sweet scent still lingered. "Of course, you think you can't bear it." She kissed me on the top of my head. "But you learn to accept it. You do."

The next morning, I arrived at the veterinary hospital the moment it opened, armed with sandwiches, a thermos of coffee, my wooden flute, and a book of poems. I had no idea how long I'd be there. Ole had stayed home, saying he'd bring the trailer if it was needed. The weekend desk clerk told me the vet was attending to another emergency, but I was welcome to go and hang out with my horse. When Buddy saw me walk in, he whinnied. He was glad to see me, but not stressed. Cash, too, seemed relaxed, as if they had both unburdened their stories during the night. Clearly they were at home with each other.

I'd brought a fold-out chair with me, and I set it up in the corner of Buddy's stall. Cash's head was at the other side of the screen. I pulled out my wooden flute and began to play quietly to the two beasts whose lives had intersected unexpectedly in the night. The horses pricked their ears and stood very still. In the large space, the notes curved in the air, then drifted up to the rafters. I played slow reels and when the music stopped the whole barn was still, as if it was waiting for something, too.

By lunchtime, Stephanie had come by to check on Buddy, and the vet had called saying she didn't have results yet but to hang in, she'd be back late afternoon. I ate one bite of sandwich and drank some coffee, drawing on all the resources I had inside me to face whatever I had to face. To calm myself, I opened a collection of poems by mystics and began to read aloud to the horses. St. Teresa of Avila, the Sufi poet Hafez, William Blake. When I got to Emily Dickinson, the horses' eyes seemed to soften:

> *In this short Life*
> *That only lasts an hour*
> *How much—how little—is*
> *Within our power*

Dickinson knew that the trajectory of our lives is a mystery: Who we meet, what changes us forever, where we end up. One moment we're trotting down a forest trail—or grazing with pals in a meadow—and next we find ourselves in a veterinary hospital with a stranger. Sometimes that connection lasts only a short, essential time. Then, in the blink of an eye, things change. Would Buddy make it through? Would Cash survive—emotionally, though he was patched up physically? Would he keep calling for his friends when he got home? There we were, three souls on a dark, December night, and very little was within our power.

It was hard to tell what time it was in that huge place. The clerestory windows in the building were way up high, but the light was fading, and soon the sound of rain pattered on the steel roof. Buddy nosed the pages as if asking for another poem. At one point he picked up the flute case and waved it in the air and dropped it in my lap. I laid my hand on his forehead, and he sighed.

The windows darkened. The vet arrived, her jacket dripping with rain. She strode in and found me in my fold-out chair, talking to my horse.

"Hello there," she said, looking me straight in the eye.

I stood up quickly. I didn't have to ask. She offered it clean and clear.

"Well," she said. "All the tests reveal that the joint sac has not been punctured at all. It looks very good." She wiped a drip of rain off her face. "And the lacerations? They'll most likely heal even faster with the injected antibiotics we gave him last night. This is the best outcome we could have asked for."

Just like that. In the blink of an eye.

Ole brought the trailer down. The vet checked Buddy's stitches, then gave his leg a clean bandage and a red leg-wrap to cover it. Christmas colors, I thought. "He can wear this for a couple days, then the smaller ones will do. He's had no lameness so you should be riding again soon. Give him a week. Ten days to be safe."

As we were finishing Buddy's final examination, Cash's owner, a middle-aged man in a jean jacket, arrived to haul him away. I could do nothing more than squeeze this man's hand an extra beat after shaking it. He eyes held mine and he said, "Thank you." He tipped his head toward Buddy. "Also, for your horse." His two sons loaded up the handsome bay who was headed for an equine rehab farm so he wouldn't have to return to an empty pasture. Neither Cash nor Buddy was alarmed at the parting, as if they had settled the business they had between them.

When Buddy was loaded safely in the trailer, I said to Ole, "I think I'll drive Buddy home tonight."

"You sure?"

I nodded. "Very sure," then hopped in the truck and turned the key.

In tandem we headed north, Ole's headlights behind us keeping my driving steady when oncoming cars whooshed by.

When we crossed the Hood Canal Bridge I clicked the windshield wipers up a notch, and thought of Mt. Olympus up there in the clouds, most likely getting mounds of snow on this winter night. My father never tired of those mountains, framing them in his drawings and photographs. He knew about composition.

When sorting through his papers, I'd recently come across a color snapshot of Lightfoot, Rosemary, and me on the Meadowdale patio. The date on the photo places me at thirteen and Rosemary nine. One shimmery branch of the birch tree is visible in the upper corner, and the shadows of a long summer evening stretch up the wide, green lawn banked by pink rhododendrons. I am sitting on a fold-out lawn chair, loosely holding Lightfoot's lead rope. Rosemary, barefoot, in a red t-shirt and shorts, is casually perched on Lightfoot's bare back—both legs hanging over his dappled left side as if she's sitting on an easy chair, hands in her lap. The house is in full sunlight, and my brother's bedroom window is open which means Paul, at fifteen, was probably reading or writing up there to get some privacy.

Dad must have taken this photo, not only because of its composition (the angles—my leaning body, Rosemary's legs, Lightfoot's neck, the shadows) but the time of day. He would have been fanning coals for a salmon on the old stone grill by the fireplace. Where was my mother? Most likely coming up the path from the kitchen with plates and salad. My parents' presence is palpable in this photograph, as if they'd only momentarily stepped out of the picture plane. All of it is gone now, of course. Meadowdale. The animals. The brief gathering of a family in time. Didn't we think it would be like that always?

As Ole's and my two-vehicle caravan pulled into town, the rain stopped. Christmas lights twinkled on the houses, and I knew I'd received the only present I could ever have asked for. I also couldn't help but feel that the whole purpose of the past twenty-four hours was for Buddy to be there for Cash. When Buddy jumped out of the trailer and danced into his paddock to meet his friends, stars glittered across the sky like broken glass.

Chapter 43.

⇾At Liberty⇽

A SPRING SUN SHINES THROUGH wispy clouds. The swallows have
returned to the barn and are making their nests with all the swoop-
ing signs of homebuilding. Buddy grazes along the far side of the
round pen. Ken hikes up his trousers and lights a smoke. "Why
don't you just get his attention? See if he's listening." I cluck, Buddy
lifts his head and comes toward my outstretched hand. I am so
proud of him doing this in front of Ken. Now that Buddy is my
horse, I am even more invested in these lessons. But at the last second, Buddy veers away and toward the grass.

"Shit," I say, my shoulders slumping.

"That's okay," Ken says. "Buddy was fine until he got distracted
by seeing me near the gate. Don't worry. Keep his attention, though.
Just bring him back. You asked him a simple thing, now make sure
you don't let go of that one little request." I cluck again and Buddy
trots away from me, wagging his head and dipping along the edges
of the ring to snatch another bite of grass.

"He's dissing you now," Ken says. "He's not afraid, he's just feeling cocky enough to say, 'Uh, I don't think so...' Which is good—
he's built so much confidence in you. But tell him you're not going
to accept that." Buddy snatches more hunks of clover like a kid

stealing from the cookie jar. "Snap the whip on the ground." Ken says. "Now!" I spank the ground and dust flies up. "Again!" Ken says.

With the second slap on the ground, Buddy takes off cantering around the ring, tossing his head. Ken moves along the outside of the rail. "You broke through his resistance just with your energy. This is good because it's *real*. You are saying to him that *you* are important. All you wanted was a simple recognition, and he chose to make a drama out of it. That's his business, but we're always looking for something quieter, more honest."

I relax my body, inviting Buddy to stop.

"He's still trotting." I so wanted to show Ken how Buddy and I had been doing amazing work in the round pen in the last few months. Leave it to expectation to get in the way.

"Buddy's a big boy, Christine. He can figure it out." Ken is right. Soon Buddy discovers I am requesting nothing more than a check-in. He slows and turns to me in the center and stops, as if to say, "So? Hey! What now?" I walk up, touch his neck, then turn away, releasing him. He wanders over to sniff a pile of manure.

"Great!" Ken says. "No drama! Buddy is clear and you are clear." I grin like a schoolgirl.

Ken reaches for his coffee on the fencepost and takes a sip. "Soon you won't need me anymore. You'll have other mentors and other experiences with Buddy—far beyond what we are doing now." He takes off his hat and scratches his short, thick hair. "You have such a great thing going with this horse. You'll be riding him around this ring naked someday." I blush (the thought of Ken picturing me naked is mildly unnerving), until I realize Ken doesn't mean me, he means riding Buddy without a saddle or bridle.

Ken adjusts his shoulders as if to loosen up the muscles Buddy was loosening. He comes out to the center of the ring and holds out his hand for me to shake it. I return the shake, but he purposely holds mine, so I can barely feel it.

"Remember, a horse doesn't want to be with someone with a limp handshake—but not a crushing one, either." Ken squeezes a bit more firmly to show the contrast. "Whether you are on the ground or in the saddle, he wants to be with someone who knows who she is. Then he can be *sure* that you are important." Ken throws his cigarette on the dirt and grinds it with his tennis shoe, then picks it up and puts it in his pocket.

"Soon, Christine, in all situations—even scary ones—he'll turn to you as the Safe Queen of the Universe." I laughed.

"Okay." Ken steps back. "Offer again what you wanted in the first place, just a polite acknowledgement." I kiss to Buddy and he turns from sniffing at the rail and, with a full friendly face, he walks toward me, eager and open. He stops right near me, I hold out my hand for a brief hello, and he touches it with his whiskers. "Beautiful," Ken says. "That's it. Connection made. Let him go. See? There's your lick and chew."

Every day with Buddy is teaching me more about how to dignify our relationship. Whether I am on Buddy's back cantering down the beach, riding in the arena practicing my balance and subtle cues, or just putting on his halter in the paddock, I am listening more and hurrying less.

A month or so after that lesson with Ken, my listening was put to the test. I was trying out a new used saddle since the one I'd been using—and considered buying from a friend—didn't fit him that well. Ole and I both had a lot more work coming in, and we decided that a well-fitted saddle for Buddy would help both him and me. Plus, Ole was talking about getting a horse for himself (Nathan!?). We began dreaming about horse camping by the Chewack River across the mountains in Eastern Washington.

I cinched up the saddle and hopped on. As I lined him out toward the edge of the forest, he was distracted, so I engaged his mind by asking him to trot in large circles with a loose rein, something we were achieving more and more. All the groundwork was really paying off. Riding was becoming an extension of our conversation on the ground. Buddy's new, elastic trot was becoming addictive, too. His back rounded out to create a cushion, as if we were both doing yoga.

When we swung counterclockwise, however, the girth loosened, and the saddle began to slip. The more the saddle listed to the left, the more agitated Buddy became. I could not right the saddle, and the more I tried to turn Buddy, my weight went with the saddle. Soon I, too, was slipping down his side.

Just as I jumped off, my boot caught in the stirrup, and the whole rig—including me—swung down Buddy's side. I felt like a trick rider, except my horse was not exactly on board with the maneuver. To him I was in the wrong place, and whatever was hanging off him now, he wanted it gone. Meanwhile I'd lost hold of the reins and quickly saw the situation unfold: me dragged all the way to Tacoma, a tattered doll beneath flailing hooves.

When I hit the ground, my leg twisted in the stirrup and I landed on my back, looking straight up at my surprised horse. Without thinking, and in the biggest, firmest, voice I could muster, I said, "WHOA!" In an instant, Buddy froze and snapped to attention, looking in astonishment at me in the grass, my leg sticking up into the awkward stirrup. The whites of his eyes were still showing, but he did not move a hair.

"Good boy," I said and slowly, slowly wrenched my boot from the stirrup, but as I came free, Buddy felt the beast on his side shift again. If that saddle started rattling under his belly, I figured I would not see him until the day after tomorrow. And while he was getting there, he'd no doubt tangle those precious legs in the rigging.

"Bud." He looked at me warily, and I slowly reached for the dangling reins. Just as I clutched them in my hand, he swung to face me, and the saddle lurched and dropped under his belly. Buddy jumped back, still not free of the enemy. Holding tight to the reins, I rose from the ground and stood tall. The kind of tall that means business.

"Buddy!" I said in my low-octave, Queen-of-the-Universe voice, giving the rein a tug to snap him out of his own drama. "You are okay. You are okay."

In an instant my horse was transformed. His eyes softened, and we both breathed a huge sigh. I wasn't just *saying* he was all right, I believed what I told him. And that made all the difference. For I did know we were both okay, and he believed it now, too. It made my heart quake with love for him, for me, for the Powers That Be. I laid my hand on his withers and told him that he'd saved us, that I was very proud. His muscles relaxed, and slowly I uncinched the renegade hunk of leather hanging underneath him, all the while talking him through it. He didn't even flinch when the saddle, like a dead cougar, finally slumped to the ground. I could hear the voice of God Herself saying to me, "You are okay." And I was.

One July evening the sky was pink, and little, puffed clouds looked like they were floating by as adornment. In summer the day keeps having extra chapters. Robins chirp until ten o'clock.

Buddy and I rode the familiar mile to the Fairgrounds, where he opened and closed the gate to the outdoor arena—a new trick we both enjoyed—and I took off all his tack and slipped on his halter and lead rope. He did a few circles, and I asked him to change directions with a tip of my head. Then I decided to risk it: I took off Buddy's halter and asked him to move around me at liberty. We weren't in the confined round pen, though. We were in the big arena where Buddy could easily bolt to the other end, just as he'd done in that first amazing lesson with Ken. But something felt right and true, so I turned my body to urge Buddy on, and he cocked his ear and trotted around me in a perfect circle. I relaxed my body and he slowed. When I picked up my energy and beamed it toward him, the circle got wider, but he didn't stray from the circle. Then I began to trot with him, my feet in step with his, my hand on his neck. The pressure was just a tiny bit too much, and he broke out of the magic bubble in one huge burst, cantering across the arena. I backed off, still feeling the connection between us. At first, I regretted that I'd chosen to work at liberty, scared he'd go bonkers and all the trust we'd built would be lost.

Until I remembered that I was his anchor now, his safe home, no matter what. I clucked quietly, stood straight as a fir tree feeling the sap rise, and held out my hand. "Buddy!" I said, my core pointing straight toward him across the arena. He spun around, perked his ears, and immediately returned to me in his elegant floating trot. Completely focused on me, he stopped—a horse-length away— and acknowledged me with a dip of his head. When I tilted my torso and asked him to make a circle around me, he tipped into the floating trot again, his neck arched, a gait as beautiful as a wave. I raised my hand and he moved into a rocking canter, one eye on me. I moved forward and he moved out; I moved back, and the circle got smaller, all the while his one ear was tuned in to me. Our bodies were attached with an invisible, pulsing thread. I could literally feel the dance.

The opening of this moment—my body speaking to Buddy's— transported me to a new language. I was finding out that when he lost his way, I had the power to invite him back. And the key word is "invite." For who wants to be forced into any relationship? With a creature, a human, or God? Isn't that one of the Great Mysteries—that we always have a choice? Every time Buddy leaves, it isn't a failure, just a new opportunity for him to return to me. In his Buddy way, he was showing me something we humans rarely access. Seduced by logic and time and words, we often miss what's actually happening. Those minutes with Buddy at the Fairgrounds offered me a glimmer of what is possible not only with a horse, but with myself and with other beings on this Earth.

Today when I arrive at Bluff Meadow on my bike, Buddy hears me coming before he sees me. His head pops up in the far field with his pals and he stops chewing, a dandelion dangling from his mouth. I put down my bike, duck under the fence, and walk out into the tall grass. "Come on, boy!" I say, and he tosses his long, white mane, swishes his tail, and canters in to see what's up. When he reaches me, I raise my arms high and ask him to rear up like Trigger, which he does with a flourish and lands calmly, bobbing his head in approval. "Thank you," I say, and we dance together in step across the meadow, his legs a perfect mirror of my own. We trot through the spongy forest path and out into the open paddock. It's only when we stop that I reach out to Buddy's nose. He touches my hand, a delicate greeting that pleases us both.

In discovering this language with my horse, I've found my own body again. Like Buddy, I resist facing ugliness and difficulty. (I still recoil thinking about Cash and his friends on the highway.) But anyone who has had to relinquish control in the face of illness, grief, or trauma knows that the body, in whatever state it's in, can be our teacher. Way back when my father gave me that lock for my bedroom closet, he gave me a physical *thing* to do for my fear of those witches. Shortly after he installed the spring latch, I'd had a dream I remember to this day: I was alone (at night, of course) on the basement stairs. As I tiptoed down in the dim light, to my horror I discovered a witch on the bottom step. All she was doing was sitting quietly, but I was utterly paralyzed. Until I did something that I cannot explain—I reached out and *touched* her wrinkly forearm. Then I looked into her eyes and saw that she, too, was a person, a being, and I said the first thing that came to my lips: "Your dress is pretty." And I believed it. I was not flattering her in order to escape; nor was I trying to buy time. Her dress actually *was* pretty with shiny black piping. And, though her face was strange and gnarled, she smiled at me—not wickedly but warmly. I was filled with power. I was no longer afraid.

My relationship with Buddy has opened a window to a deeper perception of the world. Maybe this is actually what we're called upon to do in this little life: find home in the most elemental place possible, our own skin. So when we finally shed it, it will be as natural as stepping through the gate at Bluff Meadow.

Buddy hangs out with me in the paddock while I fork knots of manure into the wheelbarrow, the fragrant piles reminders that he is alive and well, and that grass, too, is part of the great cycle of a horse's life. He sniffs the wheelbarrow, then spies my hat on the fencepost. He walks over, picks it up, and waves it around in circles. "Bring it here, Buddy. I could use a little shade," I say, and he continues waving it as he comes to me and drops it in my hand.

Some days, yes, it feels as if I'm brandishing a huge machete to beat back the sorrows of this world (which are considerable). Each time I encounter suffering, my own or others', I am incensed all over again—as if it's an aberration rather than a hard fact of being alive. I think back to when I blamed Jan Storvard for giving away the plot of *The Red Pony*. In retrospect, however, she gave me something I did not recognize in seventh grade: sooner or later, the pony is going to die, no matter what. Either in the story or beyond it. I'm beginning to see that it's not really whether the pony dies, it's how we choose to live with the news.

I kneel to scrub the water trough. Seagulls glide along the bluff and Buddy breathes on my head, his whiskers tickling the back of my neck. Instead of dropping the hose and throwing my arms around his neck like every teenage horse picture in the universe,

I continue scrubbing and dump the dirty water. "How could I be so lucky as to have you?" I ask Buddy, echoing my mother's words, knowing as she did that none of us can really "have" anything.

Then I stand up, replenishing the huge bucket with clear, fresh water. And Buddy drinks deep.

Acknowledgments

LET THE GRATITUDE BEGIN WITH my agent, Gail Hochman, who championed this memoir from the first draft. She has read every iteration since. When most agents would have stepped aside after one too many passes, she vowed to find a home for *Wild Ride Home.* Not only did she find it a home, she placed it in the expert hands of Arcade/Skyhorse's Lilly Golden, the editor of my dreams. Thank you, dear Lilly, for your keen eye, amazing instinct, and gentle care.

Some years ago, my friend and fellow poet Haas Mroue told me in no uncertain terms I must write a book about all the crazy places my poet life has taken me. So I bought a new desk and opened my laptop. But each time I tried to write about my adventures, I kept coming back to my family. I couldn't get rid of them. I finally succumbed and let them all in, still wondering who would want to read about a family like mine. As I wrote my way forward, however, I had no clue what urgent events would barge into my life—and into this narrative—demanding attention, forcing me to stop and reset the frame yet again. And again. Dearest Haas, I wish you were here to read it now.

I am hugely indebted to Sawnie Morris, "poet-on-the-couch," who, during several years of illness, read every stitch of partial chapters, ponderings. and then full drafts, saying, "Keep sending!

Keep writing!" Sas Colby, confidante and cheerleader, kept me honest. Anne Hirondelle kept me sane. Lisa Schlesinger (ah, the Bostick Trio), Dan Schmidt, Stephanie Lutgring, Bruce Bond, Billy Aronson, Dan Elish, Deborah Pedersen, Peggy Salinger (and Gus), Velma Johnson, Jo Bradley, Phil Pilgrim, David George Gordon, Erin Fristad, Rikki Ducornet, Sandy Diamond, and Marie Howe (keep paddling!) read all or parts of the manuscript in different forms. Joe Olshan, what a stroke of fortune to have received the fruits of your editing and your solid faith in the story. And Adrianne Harun, thanks for your gift of moral support and literary savvy. A nod to Ladane Nasseri for insight into Persian mystics. If I left anyone out, I offer my sincere apology and a special blessing.

Thank you, Vermont Studio Center, for a month's residency and scholarship where I met Michelle DeMarco, who painted at her easel while I read her my new chapters. Thanks also to Washington State Artist Trust for their generous Fellowship for Literature, and to the Barbara Deming Memorial Fund, Inc., for a Money for Women grant.

It's impossible to measure the ongoing intellectual, creative, and emotional sustenance I've received from my treasured friend and colleague Sands Hall. I bow to your mastery as both writer and reader. Speaking of bowing down, Mary Merralls not only read, but *listened* to all three final revisions. I sit at your feet, Mary.

And then there's Ken. Mr. Siefer, your horsemanship, friendship, and generosity have not only made me a better horseman, they've made me a better human. You showed me a new way of being that has extended into all aspects of my life. You also inspired me to find more wise teachers like yourself: Harry Whitney, Frédéric Pignon, Magali Delgado, Jessica Crouch, and Mary Anne Campbell. The writings of Klaus Hempfling and Mark Rashid have enriched my ever-expanding sense of what it means to be with a horse. I also thank my local (and faraway) horse pals who've offered me their earned wisdom. We are a fiercely loyal posse.

Now, as my niece Libby would say, "The Fam Bam!" In the spirit of Mary and Peter Hemp, I laud my siblings Paul and Rosemary, who continue to shine with constancy and love, and they've spawned the best legacy ever: Catharine! Celia! Margie! Libby! Our blazing stars! Grateful for my Norwegian mother-in-law, Lindis, who gave us Ole. Without my husband (now a notable horseman himself), I could not have pushed through this story. Along the way, I asked Ole if he might read a chapter or two. "Oh, I don't need to read it," he said. "I've lived it." He is the love of my life.

⁓ Permissions ⁓

About the Author

CHRISTINE HEMP LIVES ON WASHINGTON'S Olympic Peninsula with two horses, two cats, and one husband. She is the author of *That Fall* and has aired her essays and poetry on NPR. She teaches at the University of Iowa Summer Writing Festival and Hugo House, Seattle.